Bring It!

Bring It!

THE REVOLUTIONARY FITNESS PLAN FOR ALL LEVELS THAT BURNS FAT, BUILDS MUSCLE, AND SHREDS INCHES

TONY HORTON

WITH MAGGIE GREENWOOD-ROBINSON, PhD

RODALE

This book is in memory of and dedicated to my mom, Jean Gencarelli Horton.
Her thoughtfulness, honesty, and guidance steered me through life every step of the way.
I miss you and I love you, Mom.

—TJ

CONTENTS

PART I The Principles

If you've picked up this book, it means you probably want to make some changes to your life. It also means you are able to lift a weight (this book is heavy!). You may be worried that you're not fit enough to start this program. But don't worry about the shape you're in right now. Instead, think about the shape you'll be in later. And stop feeling guilty about neglecting your body. There's still time to show it some love. Hate exercise? Yeah, well, sometimes so do I. And if you've been working out faithfully and not seeing the results you want, don't be discouraged. No matter what shape you're in, I promise you this: My program will inspire you to find the fun in fitness and keep your body looking and feeling incredible for the rest of your life. Think of this journey as a treasure hunt where you are both the pirate explorer and the hidden prize at the end. In fact, this is the true derivation of the term *pirate's booty*, which has nothing to do with gold coins (or cheese popcorn) but, rather, the satisfaction of one's own firm glutes after repetitious climbing of the mast with a 5-pound parrot on your shoulder. (Look for this exercise in my next workout program, Pirate 90 Aaargh.)

Being healthy and fit is about more than just seeing the right number on your bathroom scale or fitting into your favorite jeans. Good health and physical fitness have powerful effects on your entire life. They will help you feel better about yourself, accomplish your goals, fulfill your intentions, and change for the better in innumerable other ways. Have you ever noticed that fit and healthy people also tend to be happy and successful? That's no coincidence. Health and success go hand in hand. (Dick Tracy: fit and successful. Homer Simpson: out of shape and miserable.) True success without good health is an illusion.

I admit that getting healthy and fit can be a challenge and requires hard work—you won't hear any superficial rah-rah speeches from me. And for many people, health and fitness prove elusive. Why? Because many of them are bamboozled and tricked by quick fixes, crazy contraptions (can you say "thigh buster"?), and gastronomic gimmicks (cabbage soup, anyone?). People love 'em. I've been in this industry for more than 25 years, and I can honestly say that if something came along to make exercise quicker and easier, I'd be all over it.

But the truth is, quick fixes don't work. That's not to say that there isn't room for innovative ideas and new exercise methods—I've tried (and stolen) plenty of good ones over the years, and I've had a hand in inventing a few. But if you're searching for the magic bullet, you'll be looking until the end of time. Because, with the rare exception of my Aunt Ethel's key lime pie and Halle Berry's cheekbones, if something seems too good to be true, well—you know the rest.

Quite often, when I share my fitness philosophy, I get a groan, a grunt, and other things that begin with *gr*. I must seem crazy to a lot of folks who were looking for a completely different answer. But I have no interest in helping you lose 10 pounds in a day or get ripped abs in 5 minutes. I am interested in your health. I care about helping you get fit, flexible, and strong. I care about helping you feel good for the rest of your life!

Many people claim they want health and happiness, yet their actions don't support their words. We give lip service to exercising more and changing our eating habits—but make no lasting changes. The national obesity rate is escalating beyond anything our health care system can handle. That is our fault—not the pharmaceutical companies', not the health care industry's, and not our government's—we've gotten lazy by eating supersized portions and fake food laced with fat, sugar, and salt and by sitting around on our collective keisters.

The way we've been living has led me to conclude that each and every one of us needs to change how we look at fitness. It's not just about dieting and exercising to make ourselves smaller. The "reason why" needs to be more profound than that. My focus has always been on feeling good, improving the quality of people's lives, being fit, and enjoying good health. Yes, I'm sure you're saying, "All that is nice, but I want to look better in a bathing suit."

Don't get me wrong: There's nothing bad about wanting to look good. I love what a fit and healthy body looks like. I'll be the first guy to show off my six-pack or flex like an Arnold wannabe. (I've already done both six times today, and I haven't even shaved yet.) But the problem is that most people exercise for the wrong reasons because they're focused solely on the outcome and not the journey. During this amazing transformation from unhealthy or moderately fit to superfit, your life will undergo several incredible changes: You'll have more energy, more opportunities, more productivity, better mental clarity, and an emotional lift from moving your body, and so much more.

One of the best examples of what I'm talking about came to me recently in the form of an e-mail from two concerned parents. Here is what they wrote.

Dear Tony,
I want to thank you for giving us our son back. For the past 15 or so years (he's 27 now), he's struggled with alcohol abuse. We tried everything we could think of to help him, and nothing worked. Then he popped in one of your P90X exercise DVDs, and the rest is history. He kept at it and stopped drinking. He started his masonry business back up again and is on top of the world. For his birthday we sent him to your fitness camp in Philadelphia, which he loved. Now the tables have turned and our son is our rock, helping us get in shape. Tony, you teach people how to get strong on the outside, but more importantly, on the inside. Thank you from the bottom of our hearts.

I live for letters and e-mails like that. Unlike physical changes, which take place gradually over time, dramatic emotional and psychological changes can happen fast. Each time you work out, eat clean whole foods, go for a hike, or get outdoors and run around, you are deliberately building a positive self-image—a physical, mental, emotional, and spiritual foundation for your growing self-esteem. The Greeks understood this principle thousands of years ago. They knew intuitively that the mind and body are one. (There are no known photos of Aristotle and Socrates, but it's common knowledge they were dead ringers for Hugh Jackman and Usher, respectively.) There's plenty of modern data to substantiate this ancient philosophy. For example, in the developing brain of a child, the impact of exercise can be long lasting because of physiologically changing and growing brain tissue. The effects are still being studied, but results show enhanced cognitive functioning, as well as improved math, logic, and reading skills, for children who get adequate exercise. Researchers are also discovering clues that vigorous exercise can stave off the beginnings of Alzheimer's disease, ADHD, and other cognitive disorders by causing older nerve cells to form dense, interconnected webs that make the brain faster and more efficient. Missing a workout is just not an option.

Keep in mind, too, that a strong, fit, and well-nourished individual will seldom feel fatigued. (Energizer Bunny: fit. Pillsbury Doughboy: easily fatigued.) Who doesn't want more energy without having to cheat to get it? By cheating, I mean alcohol, pills, potions, and processed foods. The energizing effect of a workout helps you combat notorious energy drainers such as depression, anxiety, and tension. Another explanation for the feel-good aspect of exercise, experts say, is that it provides a pleasant retreat from unpleasant thoughts, emotions, and behaviors. In that sense, exercise is similar to a relaxing hobby. It's like knitting—with sweat.

And then there's the anti-aging truth of a fit lifestyle. At the age of 52, I know that my healthy choices are saving me from the chronic pain, illness, and other suffering that many of my peers experience. It's sad to watch friends and family members become disabled by hip, back, knee, and shoulder problems; high blood pressure; type 2 diabetes; and sleep apnea—conditions that were much less prevalent just 10 years ago and which are tied to obesity and an unhealthy lifestyle. So many people who were lean and active in their twenties and thirties now face these life-crushing ailments. Old friends are turning into old men and women right before my eyes. Most of them have resigned themselves to the idea that declining health is an inevitable side effect of aging. But it's never too late to reverse the effects of aging. If you wake up every day committed to doing something to counter and prevent such ailments, you can create a happy, healthy, youthful life, no matter what your age. I've met thousands of people, from teenagers to octogenarians, who have turned their lives around. If they can do it—if *I* can do it—so can you. The first step is to believe that it can happen. I'm here to tell you that your life can improve through better, smarter choices.

How do I propose to make that happen? Let's start at the very beginning. (*A very good place to start.* C'mon, sing it with me . . .)

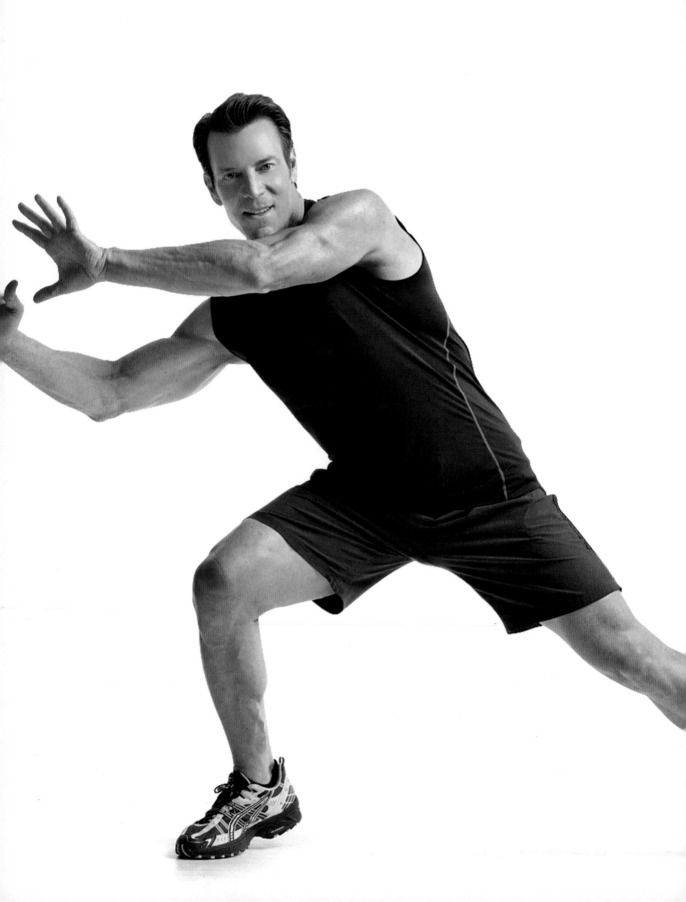

1

Feel-Good Fitness

My goal is to hand you a program with a strategy that works for you now and will continue to work for the rest of your life. That goal is achieved with a simple combination of cardiovascular exercise, resistance training, and flexibility work, combined with healthy eating. It's not a complicated plan. The people I work with want simplicity and results, and that's what you'll get here.

The plan I'm offering you is the same one I do myself. I work out with free weights, body weight, and resistance bands for 45 to 55 minutes 2 or 3 days a week at my home. Biceps curls, shoulder presses, lunges, situps, and pushups, plus a healthy dose of unusual exercises (you'll learn them here!), will challenge your balance, flexibility, core strength, and endurance. And ladies, speaking of pushups, for those of you who claim you can't do a standard pushup, I'll have you doing at least 10 before you finish this book! For cardio, I do 45 to 50 minutes 2 days a week, with as many different types of aerobic moves as I can cram into that time period. Yoga and stretching are musts for me, as is a hard-core plyometric interval routine that hammers my legs and glutes.

One of the main reasons why I stay fit is so that I can participate in the sports I love. Every Sunday morning, I head down to the original Muscle Beach near my home in Santa Monica, California, to meet up with a group of friends for an outdoor gymnastics session. We turn basic pullups, pushups, and situps into a much more intense combination of plyometric pullups, swing hand-stands, and 25-foot rope climbs (hands only and upside down), plus isometric core exercises. We even throw in a backflip or two.

On an occasional Wednesday night, I meet up with a group to go rock climbing. Every fall, I get together with ski buddies and work on ways to get our legs ready for the slopes. To me, there's nothing better than the great outdoors. The sports I enjoy most involve clean air, gorgeous views, and climbing up or ripping down pristine mountains. I also try to mix in other activities like in-line skating, table tennis, basketball, and mountain biking. When I'm at the beach or skiing, I'm one with my surroundings, happy as a clam and at peace with life. Participating in sports is a fun way to enjoy a healthy, active lifestyle. (Note to self for next book: Find out if clams are really happy. If an active lifestyle is the secret to happiness, consider using the phrase "happy as a hummingbird.")

And so, the program in this book is built around what I do—and what I know works, based on the results of thousands of men and women who have experienced amazing life changes using my programs. This program revolves around four key principles.

PRINCIPLE # I: Individualization

A big reason why so many people have trouble staying on track is that they get caught up in the latest trend and don't focus on what they need as individuals. Your fitness choices should play to your "exercise personality." (We all have one, even if it has never been tapped into.) You may be someone who hates exercise, but you know you need to get moving. Gyms intimidate you. You think sweating is gross, and you've never had an athletic day in your life. Or maybe you're someone who exercises sporadically and the results have come at a snail's pace, if at all. Yes, I'm sure you have a ton of good excuses as to why your workouts have been hit or miss, but I can counter with a million more good reasons to be consistent—one of the most important being how you think and feel every day of the week, not just once in a while.

Maybe you're someone who loves to exercise, but you don't have the right formula. Chances are you've been wasting money on gym memberships and trainers who aren't giving you the results you've been looking for. You feel as if you've been doing everything "right," but you're frustrated by your lack of progress. I will show you how you can save tons of time, money, and energy by getting the best workouts possible right in your own home.

Perhaps the pleasures—and the benefits—have been lost on you because you've had nothing but negative experiences with working out and dieting. In my work as a trainer, I've found that many people exercise for the wrong reasons, or they don't do what's right for them, so they give up. Whether you're a busy mom with only minutes to spare or an athlete looking for peak performance, you will find something in this program to fit your needs and meet your goals. You see, exercise isn't a one-size-fits-all prescription. I design unique fitness programs for each person I train. Just pumping out generic workouts won't cut it. If I create a fitness program customized for a client's individual fitness preferences, physical condition, goals, and lifestyle, the odds are he or she will stay motivated and stick with it. Motivation is huge in helping you stay committed to this program so that positive long-term lifestyle changes can happen. When you choose the fitness program designed for your personality, you'll get excited about your potential.

PRINCIPLE #2: Periodization Training

We all need some excitement in our lives. When it comes to working out, we tend to appreciate familiarity and remain loyal to what works for us, but it's important to venture outside of our comfort zones and try different things that offer different benefits. The same principle applies to our relationships, work situations, and other choices in life. Well, I can't tell you how to heat up your love life (not in this book anyway), but in terms of exercise, if you've been training for a while and your progress has stopped or your workouts have gotten stale, I will certainly put some zing back into your training (which will make it *trainzing*?).

Anytime you present your body with a new physical challenge, it starts to respond in positive ways almost immediately. But when you do a physical task repeatedly, your body figures out a way to become more efficient and expends less energy. The result? The dreaded plateau. Your body will naturally stall as your fitness routine becomes second nature. This is what many people experience with traditional fitness programs: Your exercise sequence leads to a stalemate—no more growth, an increased risk of injuries, and less fat-burning.

Well, there will be no plateaus here—only continual, nonstop progress. Here's why: Each workout in this book incorporates some form of *periodization training*.

Periodization training doesn't sound like your typical workout term. It sounds more like a grammar rule you never bothered to memorize in fourth-grade English class. Put succinctly, periodization training is a protocol designed to avoid plateaus and produce continued gains. Your body will typically adjust to the specific stress you give it, but varying your regimen through periodization training forces it to adapt again and grow in the process. If you want a new or continued adaptation, you must do something new or continually add a different type of stress to your system.

Periodization training makes that happen by manipulating five fitness variables: volume, cycles, intensity, frequency, and active rest.

Volume is how much time you spend exercising aerobically or the load of weight lifted (dumbbells, bands, or body weight) multiplied by repetitions. You'll be changing up your volume as you progress through each workout. And no, you won't need a calculator or degree in algebra.

Cycles describe sections of your workout—specifically, macro-cycles and micro-cycles. A macro-cycle in this book lasts 6 weeks and is broken down into weekly training emphases (micro-cycles). The goal of the macro-cycle is to maximize adaptation and thus prevent plateaus. Basically, you'll advance from easier workouts that use lighter weights to progressively heavier weights and more reps per exercise set. Unlike traditional exercise programs, which either keep the repetitions the same throughout the year or may go through different rep ranges in one workout, periodization training alters resistance and rep considerations. These regular changes not only provide differing emphases on your muscles but also keep your enthusiasm up and boredom at bay.

Intensity is the level of effort you put forth. During cardio training, working out at a particular percentage of your heart rate is an indicator of intensity. In resistance training, intensity can be determined by working with maximum load for a certain number of repetitions.

Frequency is a darn good movie with Dennis Quaid. It also refers to the number of training sessions per day, week, or month. For example, the old standard has been 3 days per week, but I'm going to show you the benefits of working out most days of the week, starting with 20 minutes a day and progressing to 55 minutes a day.

Active rest is not a time of inactivity but a transition period that allows the body to rest before it begins another micro-cycle of training. Active rest includes physical activities that pump up the fun, such as sports, cycling, swimming, dance, and yoga. In the next chapter, I'll help you identify the activities that are the best fit for you.

With periodization training, you'll learn how to make your muscles do unexpected and unfamiliar things, or familiar things in unexpected ways so that you keep burning fat and your fitness curve continues to climb skyward. You'll learn how to continually challenge your muscles into responding—the secret behind getting results. Your body doesn't respond to repetition; it responds to novelty. Often, people assume the key to persevering is to master one or two workouts, when, in fact, monotony is often a huge reason for failure. I advocate variety: Shake it up and do something different every day. You want it, I've got it: cardio, strength, flexibility, balance work, belly and core exercises, and plenty of muscle sculpting. It's all in here. It's a form of physical chess. Your body doesn't know what's coming next and is constantly stimulated to change and forced to adapt to that change. Boredom and injuries are eliminated because volume, cycles, intensity, frequency, and active rest won't let them happen.

And instead of working each body part individually, like many other workout programs suggest, I combine exercises so you get an all-in-one body-toning, muscle-sculpting, fat-burning workout. Think of it as multitasking for your muscles.

In addition, your body will constantly face new challenges. This workout is not about simply checking off boxes and advancing from one level to the next. In fact, it's a little like rock climbing—filled with challenging, ever-changing "terrain" and surprises. The unfamiliarity of a variety of different exercise techniques will help your body burn fat continuously, stimulate new muscle growth, protect connective tissue, prevent boredom, and get you into the best shape of your life. A vast majority of my moves and exercises are extreme and dynamic—nothing is stale or boring, I promise. I'll give you the most effective, varied routines imaginable, regardless of whether you have an hour or just 20 minutes to devote to exercise. Even if you hate exercise now, you're going to develop a true passion for fitness.

PRINCIPLE #3: Progression

The exercise personality test in Chapter 2 will help you figure out your current fitness level and the program best suited to your needs. I've designed workouts for three levels of fitness: Beginners, Strivers, and Warriors. No matter which program you select, you'll see improvements in how you feel and look *within the first week.* That's because I'm going to give you a unique three-tiered program, with specific strategies to help you advance your fitness level.

Each program contains core conditioning, cardio workouts, interval training, resistance training, and flexibility exercises. You'll progress within each of these workouts, starting with Phase 1 routines and moving right up to more intense Phase 2 routines. If you're a Beginner, I'll show you how to move up to Striver and ultimately to Warrior. Same goes for Strivers; you'll progress to a Warrior. If you start as a Warrior, you'll experience the kind of results you've been dreaming about. This three-tiered approach is great for everyone, from first timers to highly advanced fitness buffs. The secret is simple: Change the routines, amp up the intensity, and bask in the results. As your overall level of health and fitness improves, so will your physique, mood, strength, flexibility, balance, and self-esteem.

If you follow this program as I've designed it, you'll discover something very powerful: **You are tougher than you think!** This is the number one piece of feedback I get from people who buy my DVDs and attend my fitness camps and seminars. It turns out that a lot of folks aren't giving their all. The truth is, people aren't seeing results because they barely put in 50 percent, let alone 110.

Take Brian, for example. At the age of 45, he'd spent most of his life being obese and unhappy. He'd tried every fad diet and gimmick imaginable, only to experience temporary success. "I shouldn't even call it success," he told me. "I should call it failure, because I always ended up heavier than when I started." Sadly, one of the "gimmicks" Brian tried was the fen-phen drug combination, popular in the early 1990s. It caused so much damage to his heart that he was able to receive compensation from a class-action lawsuit filed against the drug company.

By October 2008, Brian tipped the scales at 308 pounds. Disgusted with himself, he cleaned up his diet and was able to lose some of the weight. But he soon hit a plateau and wasn't losing a pound or an inch. Brian considered trying P90X but feared that it would be "too intense." He overcame his reluctance and bought it anyway. He struggled a little when he started out and made plenty of modifications to suit his fitness level, but within 4 short months (during which he progressed to more challenging routines), Brian stripped off another 102 pounds and now weighs in at a fit

185 pounds. And there's more to his story: Brian reports that he's now in "awesome health"—no more high blood pressure and no more joint pain. Brian, like most people, learned that he was tougher than he'd ever imagined.

PRINCIPLE #4: Cleanse-Nourish-Supplement

My eating plan places an emphasis on foods that make you feel good and look good; that is, they boost energy, enhance immunity, promote mental clarity, brighten mood, and improve general health. These very same foods will also help you look your best; they keep your body's fat-burning process going 24/7 while simultaneously supporting the growth of long, lean muscle and promoting healthy, glowing skin, hair, and other aspects of your outer appearance.

You'll learn how to change your nutritional habits in my three-part Meal Plan. Part 1 cleanses toxins like caffeine, alcohol, and processed foods from your diet, and Part 2 replaces them with nourishing whole foods. Those foods include natural carbohydrates and lean proteins, which fuel your neuromuscular system and prime fat metabolism. These carb-rich health foods, coupled with training, will maximize your energy stores and work capacity. You'll also eat lean protein to help develop and maintain body-firming muscle mass. And you'll replace all of the unhealthy fats you've been eating with healthy ones, which are vital to your body's functioning as they provide energy, nutrient transport, and storage, as well as structure, protection, and insulation for your hormones

Avoid "Exercise Bipolar Disorder"!

I encourage you to move your body most days. Doing so will help you avoid what I call exercise bipolar disorder, or EBD. When you exercise, your brain increases the output of feel-good chemicals like dopamine, norepinephrine, serotonin, and adrenaline. These chemicals stay elevated in your brain for about 24 hours—longer than most mood drugs last. Working out regularly provides a steady stimulus to your muscles and mind, resulting in continued physical strength and mental well-being. On the other hand, if you work out on Monday and skip Tuesday, by the time Wednesday rolls around you could be in a full frontal funk—because those feel-good chemicals are gone.

The "cure" for EBD is to move your body 5 to 7 days a week to keep these chemicals naturally elevated. This may seem like a lot to take on, but trust me, you can do it. People write to me all the time saying, "I started your program wanting to look better, but I am sticking with it because of the way I feel" or "I started because I wanted to lose a dress size, but I stay with it because I'm a better mom" or "I got into this because I wanted the numbers on the scale to go down, but now I'm hooked because I have the enthusiasm to try things I have never done before." When you move your body, you heal your mind.

and cells. In Part 3, I'll provide an overview of supplements and give you science-backed guidance on which supplements will work best for you.

By starting my program, you commit to a lifestyle that honors the innate wisdom that comes from within your body and your mind. If you have concerns regarding your weight, remind yourself that at its proper weight, your body will feel buoyant and agile, and your brain will operate at its peak mental clarity and emotional resilience. Your newfound vitality will become a source of joy and motivation in your life. What a gift that this type of fitness and happiness can be achieved by anybody, regardless of age, gender, lifestyle, or financial level—and requires no special effort outside of moving your body and satisfying your hunger with nourishing, wholesome foods.

I believe that the root of authentic joy and happiness is how you treat your body. One thing you can be sure of is that life will challenge you, calling upon your physical, mental, and emotional resources in ways you can't imagine. A fit body and mind empower you to handle whatever life throws your way. Don't wait any longer—choose to live a life of freedom, health, and abundant energy now.

The Bring It! Edge

When you follow the program in this book, you will not only lose weight, you'll also get healthier. Expect to experience any (or all!) of the following benefits:

- Cardiovascular endurance
- More energy
- Increased muscle tone
- Less body fat
- Lower blood pressure and resting heart rate
- Lower cholesterol
- Less stress and anxiety
- Mood and attitude booster
- Better sleep

- Increased mental alertness and clarity
- Improved memory function
- Higher self-esteem
- Better goal-setting processes
- A greater sense of hope, joy, and optimism
- Improved penmanship (not really—just want to make sure you're still paying attention)

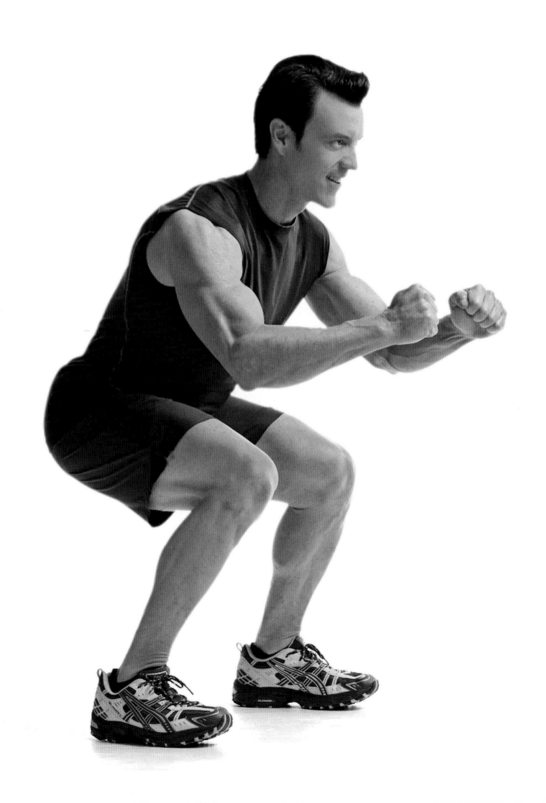

2

What's Your FQ?

Before you lace up your cross trainers and start

sweating with me, let's sit down together and figure out a little bit more about your current state of fitness. Up until now, many of you have been working out sporadically; others of you have been avoiding the gym for years. You might be someone who wants to lose weight but hasn't been seeing results from your current exercise routine. Or maybe you're already pretty fit but you want to take your fitness to a whole new level.

To help you take your next step (or perhaps your first), I've created a fitness assessment called the Fitness Quotient (FQ) test. Relax, this test doesn't contain trick questions or require a No. 2 pencil, and I won't grade you on your results. You're about to explore your inner fitness guru: your motivation, body image, preferences, and desires—the whole shebang—and your physical capacity to become more active and fit. (And while you do that, I'm going to explore why I used the word *shebang* and whether I should worry about accidentally breaking out *zowie* or *cowabunga* in future chapters.)

This test is meant to steer you on the right course to lifelong fitness. What you'll learn from your score could mean the difference between successful, long-term wellness and a fitness flop. Your truthful answers to these questions will help us create a fitness plan specifically for YOU. Herein lies the magic that will keep you motivated as you see and feel increased endurance, strength, balance, and flexibility. Let's figure out how to get you started.

My Fitness Quotient is divided into two parts. Part 1 is designed to pinpoint your level of conditioning and motivation. Your answers will guide you to the right workout plan for your lifestyle.

Part 2 will help you find your *fun factor*—the kinds of activities I'd like you to engage in during your active rest time. What is playful, challenging, and interesting to you? Participating in sports and recreational activities that you enjoy will keep you motivated and help you develop balance, endurance, and coordination—which accelerate your results. I want you to ski, dance, skate, ride, run, ping, pong, and play!

Be a child again, or try being childlike for the first time. Young children have a freedom associated with everything they do. They don't care who's watching, what people think, or the consequences of any of their silliness. They are active and engaged in the moment without judgments of any kind. Exercise shouldn't feel like ditch digging or rocket science—it's supposed to be fun. Your answers to the FQ will show you how to create a fitness routine that you can actually look forward to doing.

So grab your pen or pencil, and let's go. Better yet, grab your crayon, kiddo.

PART 1: Find Your Fitness Level

Read each question or statement thoroughly. Choose "a," "b," or "c," depending on how the answer best reflects you. Answer each question as honestly as you can. If in doubt, go with your gut.

1. Which statement most accurately describes your exercise history?
   a. I've always exercised consistently, pushing myself to get better and better.
   b. I've always done some sort of exercise, but I haven't always been consistent.
   c. I've tried different types of exercises, but I've never stuck with any of them.

2. How long has it been since you participated in regular exercise?
   a. I'm currently exercising.
   b. It's been 2 months or more.
   c. When was Carter president?

3. How many pushups do you think you can do?
   a. More than 30.
   b. 8 to 12.
   c. Zero to 5 or a few more—on my knees. And at gunpoint.

4. How would you describe your flexibility; for example, can you touch your toes easily?
   a. My middle name is Gumby.
   b. I'm almost there.
   c. Ouch!

5. How many sports do you play?

   a. 4 to 8.

   b. 1 or 2.

   c. Is watching *American Idol* a sport?

6. How would you describe your physical status?

   a. Very fit.

   b. Fairly fit.

   c. I have other beautiful qualities once you get to know me.

7. How physically strong are you?

   a. I have no problem carrying groceries and luggage, shoveling snow, or doing strenuous chores around the house.

   b. I can lift moderately heavy objects, but sometimes I must strain to do it.

   c. Lifting things? Chores? Is this a question for my cleaning lady?

8. How often do you choose stairs over elevators or escalators?

   a. Every time.

   b. Occasionally.

   c. Why would someone do that?

9. Identify your response to the following statement: "I would feel a real loss if I were forced to give up exercising."

   a. An emphatic YES!

   b. I agree somewhat.

   c. Not so much.

10. How many hours a day do you watch television?

    a. None to 2.

    b. 3 to 4.

    c. The one in my living room or the one in my bedroom?

11. Do you consider yourself overweight?

    a. No.

    b. A little; maybe 5 to 15 pounds.

    c. Yes, 15 pounds or more.

12. Do you get enough satisfying sleep?

    a. Always.

    b. Sometimes.

    c. I can't answer because I just fell asleep taking this test.

13. Do you feel comfortable in a gym or when engaging in athletic activities?

  a. Most of the time.

  b. Sometimes.

  c. It brings back too many painful memories, many of which involve dodgeball.

14. Did you participate in athletics as a child?

  a. All the time.

  b. Sporadically.

  c. Can we stop talking about the dodgeball?

15. How do you feel when you think about physical activity?

  a. I get fired up.

  b. I need a nudge.

  c. I would rather chew on plastic.

16. What is your perceived intensity (level of effort) when exercising?

  a. Like a bull in the ring.

  b. Like the average bear.

  c. Like the average bear—in hibernation.

17. Have you ever had any negative feelings or experiences associated with exercising?

  a. Rarely.

  b. Sometimes.

  c. Again with the dodgeball?

18. When stressful or difficult situations arise, you:

  a. Exercise anyway and use my workout for stress relief.

  b. Make an effort to exercise but sometimes blow it off.

  c. Opt out of exercising because I'm too anxious or stressed-out to consider it.

19. Which of the following statements generally describes your attitude about exercise?

  a. I like to start or end my day with a workout.

  b. I tend to go with the flow. If I feel like exercising before or after work, I will. If I don't, I won't.

  c. I'm usually tired after a day at work. I can't think of anything but going home and putting my feet up.

20. How do you feel about your body?

  a. I'm very comfortable with my body and not afraid to try new ways of working out.

  b. I'm fairly comfortable with my body, but I know there's room for improvement.

  c. I don't like my body very much; I don't feel comfortable with it.

21. Do you feel self-conscious wearing a bathing suit in public?

    a. Not usually.

    b. Sometimes.

    c. I would sooner wear my Batman costume to church on Easter Sunday.

22. If you pass by a mirror and see your reflection, what do you say?

    a. Look at my reflection! Now look at me! Now my reflection! Now back to me!

    b. Time to step it up, Bucko. (And don't ever call me Bucko again.)

    c. Why is there a circus mirror in my house?

23. Have you ever been told by your physician that you have exercise restrictions due to heart trouble, arthritis, diabetes, or another physical condition?

    a. No.

    b. On occasion.

    c. Yes, I have a chronic condition and have to be careful.

24. How would you describe your diet?

    a. I have a loving and healthy relationship with vegetables and legumes.

    b. I do okay.

    c. I'm familiar with the Golden Arches.

25. How often do you eat starchy foods (bread, pasta, cereal, etc.) and sweets (candy, desserts, sugar, etc.)?

    a. Never to rarely.

    b. Occasionally.

    c. Do I get a chocolate croissant for finishing this test so quickly?

Scoring

Add up the number of "a" answers, "b" answers, and "c" answers, and score yourself according to the following key.

Mostly A's:

Fitness level: Warrior. You enjoy physical activity and work out consistently. Exercise was probably part of your natural routine in childhood. You are self-motivated and fairly disciplined, and you enjoy working out several times a week. You like your body and are confident in the way it performs. You may, however, find yourself falling into a fitness rut that could lead to burnout or injury. You need something new. Follow the exercise and dietary guidelines designed for *Warriors* (see page 73). Also, your lucky number is pi, and your lucky color is mauve.

Mostly Bs:

Fitness level: Striver. Physical activity is not foreign to you, but chances are, if you've ever joined a gym or an athletic league, you quit early on because you grew frustrated or bored. You need more consistency in your fitness program. But by taking this quiz, you've shown you are interested in changing your patterns—and making fitness a part of your life. Follow the exercise and dietary guidelines designed for *Strivers* (see page 61). Your lucky number is the square root of 6. Famous Strivers include Maria and her parents, Eunice and Sargent Striver.

Mostly Cs:

Fitness level: Beginner. You see yourself as an exercise "outsider" and often get overwhelmed at the thought of working out. You're honest enough to admit that you're among the majority of Americans who, while not necessarily sedentary, aren't doing enough physical activity to improve their health. The fact that you've picked up this book is a great step in the right direction. You know you need to get healthy, though. To begin improving your health, fitness, and self-image, follow the exercise and dietary guidelines designed for *Beginners* (see page 47). Your lucky number is negative 4, and your lucky day is—today.

In the Middle:

In some cases, you might find yourself between Beginner and Striver, or Striver and Warrior. If so, start with the lower level. Should you discover that you need more of a challenge, take it up a notch to either Striver or Warrior.

If you've scored as a Beginner, don't beat yourself up. The progress you'll make in just 3 weeks will be phenomenal, and if you stick with it, you'll be a Striver in no time. Let me share a story. Chris, a 37-year-old mother, started this program as a 30-pounds-overweight Beginner and self-proclaimed couch potato. "I was struggling to pick up my little girl, who is the absolute joy in my life," says Chris, who had also been diagnosed with high cholesterol.

Chris stayed faithful to the Beginner's program and experienced incredible results. In her words: "My doctor was shocked when he saw my cholesterol numbers drop by half. I can get into my 'skinny jeans.' And not only can I pick up my daughter with ease, I don't want to put her down!"

Get excited, Beginners! Your life is about to change.

PART 2: Find Your Fun Factor

The key to sticking with any exercise program is finding fun activities that keep you interested and motivated. Now that you've identified your fitness level, read through the following profiles to help you identify your fun factor—activities that will help you get and stay fit but that feel more like play than exercise.

Check any and all boxes that best describe you. Your choices will direct you to the kinds of fun activities you'll enjoy and stick with.

Meditative Player

- ☐ I enjoy activities that relax my body, mind, and spirit.
- ☐ My idea of a perfect vacation is a spiritual pilgrimage.
- ☐ I like exercise that involves slow, deliberate movements that bring perfect harmony to my mind and body.
- ☐ Puttering in my garden and taking my dog on a hike are some of my favorite activities.
- ☐ I prefer solo exercise activities to group activities.

Social Player

- ☐ I like group fitness classes. I feed off the energy of the music and the motivation of the instructor.
- ☐ I prefer hanging out with friends to spending time alone.
- ☐ I like activities in which anyone can participate, even someone who has never done them before.
- ☐ I dance however I like, without worrying about how I look.
- ☐ I prefer activities in which skill level doesn't matter. It's all about having a fun experience.

Team Player

- ☐ I root for sports teams, not individual players.
- ☐ I have enjoyed playing team sports such as basketball, softball, or baseball.
- ☐ I feel comfortable participating in group activities.
- ☐ I participated in team sports as a kid and really enjoyed it.
- ☐ After a hard week at work, I can't wait to meet my friends for a pickup basketball game or a run with a runners' club, of which I am a member.

Extreme Player

- ☐ The idea of snowboarding or snow biking appeals to me.
- ☐ Given a choice, I'd rather exercise outside.
- ☐ I feel energized by activities involving elements of danger or physical risk.

☐   I enjoy pursuing some of the coolest new sports fads.

☐   I like to be active, mostly for the rush it brings.

Competitive Player

☐   I sometimes look for ways to show that I can outshine others.

☐   Getting my competitive juices flowing makes my workout more enjoyable.

☐   I like engaging in competitive forms of recreation, such as races or contests (especially if I win).

☐   I prefer to compete in individual sports, such as running, bicycling, or swimming.

☐   My favorite pastime is anything that's competitive.

Recommendations

Meditative Player. You seek inner stillness and peace and enjoy solitary activities. Adding a yoga class, Pilates, tai chi, or simple stretching to my program will bring you relief from the physical and mental pressures of a busy day. You may crave quiet time for yourself while you exercise. Running, swimming, and cycling are all great solo activities. Try bicycle Spinning classes, which require serious focus, or take a Zen-like approach to the exercise routines in this book and do them alone, in a quiet room or empty house (kimono optional).

Social Player. You're the kind of person who loves to be with others and finds physical activity to be most enjoyable when shared with significant people in your life. The time spent laughing with others and sharing your life makes the exercise sessions go by quickly. As you follow my program, consider asking a friend or workout buddy to join you.

To boost your fun factor, supplement my program with activities such as dance fitness classes (Latin fusion, hip-hop, step aerobics, ballet, and so forth). Try engaging in active social pastimes as well, such as in-line skating or cycling with friends, playing tennis, or taking a sailing or rock climbing class. My friend Scotty Fifer recommends flying trapeze class.

Team Player. You're also very social, craving laughter, excitement, and togetherness. You like being part of a team and sharing your successes. Try joining a softball league or playing soccer or beach volleyball. Feel free to audition for the Olympic curling team.

Extreme Player. On the track, field, court, or mat, you're a no-holds-barred person who gives it your all. You love to get your adrenaline pumping with the latest sports craze. You enjoy exercising outdoors, breathing fresh air, and you get excited over new things and thrive on change. Check out activities like waterskiing, kayaking, scuba diving, snowboarding, mountain biking, or surfing. This is the category I fit in, by the way!

Competitive Player. Your natural athleticism lets you choose from a variety of team and individual sports, as well as competitive endurance sports, such as marathons or triathlons. Because you tend to be competitive, try martial arts and work your way up the belt colors in karate. Call me when you get to chartreuse.

Here's something else I need to squeeze in. Maybe you used to play sports, recreational or otherwise, but being out of shape put those activities on hold. Not anymore. Once you get back in shape, you'll be able to resume your favorite activities again and put more fun into your life. That's exactly what happened to Ron. He had been an avid skier since age 16. But an unhealthy lifestyle and the resultant excessive weight took its toll. No longer could he enjoy his favorite sport. Once he tried to go skiing but could barely manage one run, while his ski buddies watched. "The humiliation I felt pushed me over the edge," Ron confessed. "I decided to change my life." Ron started P90X and regained his aerobic and muscular endurance. He's back on the slopes. "Skiing is now a joy again," he says.

The people who stick with exercise for the long haul are those who enjoy it. They do it out of fun and interest and because it's a challenge. These are people who will continue exercising long after they lose 10 or 30 pounds. So choose activities that fit your approach to life—and you'll stay fit for life.

Now there's one more test to take. This time, you can put on your gym shoes and workout clothes. Go ahead, I won't peek.

Tony's Motivators: "Curiosity Killed the Rut"

This is a phrase I often use. It means I want you to be curious about new fitness techniques. If you're in a fitness slump now, or you fall into one in the future, it's probably because you've been doing the same thing for a long time and you're bored. Worse, you're not seeing any real change, nor are you getting better.

The cure is curiosity. It leads to experiences you would never have otherwise discovered. Say, for example, you're curious about rock climbing. Go to a rock climbing gym. Or if that doesn't appeal to you, try something you've never done before, such as mountain biking, a Spinning class, kayaking, or yoga.

You can also try different instructors. I go to different yoga instructors all the time, for example. Each one has a different style, different sequences, and different moves. Each time that you do something different, you learn something new and improve your balance, coordination, and stamina. And most importantly, you keep your brain engaged and interested.

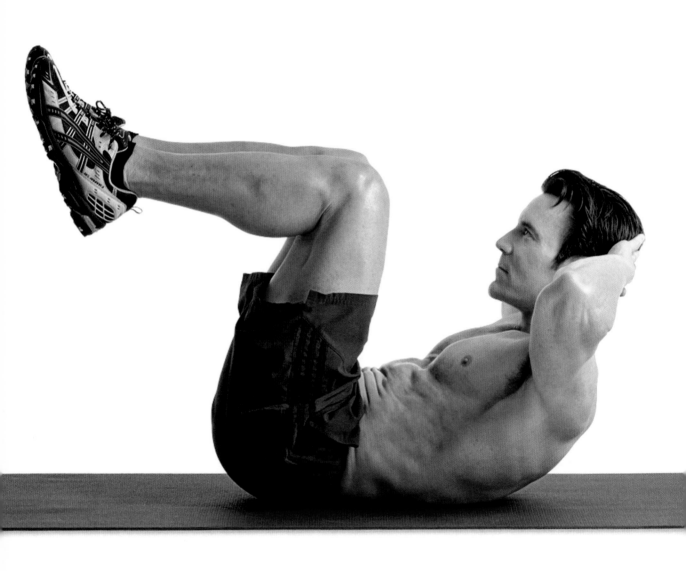

3

How Fit Are You?

Short of hiring a personal trainer to evaluate

your condition, you can only guess where your physical strengths—and weaknesses—may lie. I have a solution. My Fit Test rates your actual ability, just like a trainer would. In this chapter, I'll show you how to gauge your cardiovascular capacity, body composition, flexibility, and muscular strength and endurance.

If the thought of a physical fitness test brings back bad memories from gym class, don't worry. You can't fail this test. Rather, think of it as a tool to help you improve your fitness and health. You'll be benchmarking yourself, and as you consistently follow my program, you'll see noticeable improvement in your scores, and you'll start to feel more energized and confident about your physical abilities.

That is exactly what happened to 35-year-old Delilah, an active-duty soldier in the U.S. Army. Delilah took a similar fitness test called the Army Physical Fitness Test (APFT), administered to all soldiers in the U.S. Army twice a year. The 300-point test is composed of three timed segments, each worth 100 points: a 2-mile run, a 2-minute pushup drill, and a 2-minute situp test. A score is determined using a standardized table that compares the soldier's age and gender to the running time in minutes and the number of completed situps and pushups. Soldiers are required to score a minimum of 60 points on each event in order to graduate Army Basic Training.

Prior to doing P90X, Delilah, at 5 foot 6, weighed 160 pounds with 27 percent body fat, and she huffed and puffed her way through the APFT. Although she met the minimum standards, she wanted to do better so she could go far in the military—the right attitude for success in almost any job. The next time she had to take the test, Delilah was ready. She had lost 20 pounds on my program and stripped her body fat down to 13 percent. She not only met the maximum standard (300 points) for her age and gender, she surpassed them, scoring an amazing 345 points. Delilah can do 67 pushups in 2 minutes and 109 situps in 2 minutes, and she can run the 2 miles flat out in 13:45. Not only that, she's now competing in half marathons and raves that she's in "the best shape" of her life. "I look better than when I was 18," she says. "I am stronger and healthier, and some nagging knee and back problems I had are gone."

Taking my Fit Test is an easy exercise that can help you get a quick fix on just how fit you really are—and on how much added effort it will take to get into peak condition. Here's the plan: Do each part of the test. Record your results. Stick to my program, and then test yourself every 4 to 6 weeks. And, merely by taking the test, you get an A for making an effort to improve your fitness.

Cardiovascular Fitness

TEST: Resting Heart Rate

One thing health care professionals have always known is that you can tell a lot about a person's health based on his or her resting heart rate (RHR), the number of times your heart beats in 1 minute when you are at complete rest. Physically fit individuals tend to have lower RHRs, indicating that their health is typically better. A high RHR is indicative of poor health and may even signal a higher risk of death from a cardiac event. So in general, the more fit you are, the stronger your heartbeat, and the more blood you pump with each beat.

How to Find Your RHR: Just before you get out of bed in the morning, sit quietly for 5 minutes, then take your pulse. Turn one hand palm up and, with the tips of your other index and middle finger, gently press the pulse point on the wrist just below the base of the thumb. Feel over your radial artery until you feel a beat. Then count the number of heartbeats for 1 minute. That's your pulse rate. Record the number of beats per minute (bpm) and the date; do this for 3 consecutive days and take an average of the three.

What Your Results Mean: A normal resting heart rate is defined by the American Heart Association as between 60 and 80 bpm. (Unless you're a great whale [7 bpm] or a shrew [800 bpm], and if you are either of those, kudos on learning how to read.) As can be seen in the chart on the opposite page, your RHR can vary with your fitness level, and with age. The good news is that a high RHR can be lowered through physical activity. Exercise improves the function of the autonomic nervous system, which controls basic body functions such as heart rate and blood pressure.

As quickly as 1 week after starting a *consistent* exercise program, expect a drop of about 1 beat per minute in your RHR (which means your heart muscle is already getting stronger and pumping more blood with each beat). After a month, there will be a total drop of about 4 beats per minute in your RHR. After about 3 months, your RHR will drop, on average, another 5 to 7 beats.

Men

AGE	18–25	26–35	36–45	46–55	56–65	66+
ATHLETE	49–55	49–54	50–56	50–57	51–56	50–55
EXCELLENT	56–61	55–61	57–62	58–63	57–61	56–61
GOOD	62–65	62–65	63–66	64–67	62–67	62–65
ABOVE AVERAGE	66–69	66–70	67–70	68–71	68–71	66–69
AVERAGE	70–73	71–74	71–75	72–76	72–75	70–73
BELOW AVERAGE	74–81	75–81	76–82	77–83	76–81	74–79
POOR	82+	82+	83+	84+	82+	80+

SOURCES: MEDLINEPLUS, AMERICAN HEART ASSOCIATION, HEALTHFINDER.GOV

Women

AGE	18–25	26–35	36–45	46–55	56–65	66+
ATHLETE	54–60	54–59	54–59	54–60	54–59	54–59
EXCELLENT	61–65	60–64	60–64	61–65	60–64	60–64
GOOD	66–69	65–68	65–69	66–69	65–68	65–68
ABOVE AVERAGE	70–73	69–72	70–73	70–73	69–73	69–72
AVERAGE	74–78	73–76	74–78	74–77	74–77	73–76
BELOW AVERAGE	79–84	77–82	79–84	78–83	78–83	77–84
POOR	85+	83+	85+	84+	84+	84+

SOURCES: MEDLINEPLUS, AMERICAN HEART ASSOCIATION, HEALTHFINDER.GOV

TEST: Stepups

Here's where you'll measure your working heart rate—the level at which you want your heart to beat to ensure you are working at an aerobic pace. Generally speaking, you want to work at a rate that is 75 to 80 percent of your maximal heart rate. Maximal heart rate per minute is found by subtracting your age from 220. I'm 52, so my maximal heart rate would be 168.

To get your working heart rate range (also called your training zone), multiply your maximal heart rate by 0.75 and 0.80. Using myself as an example again, my range would be 126 to 134. A quick way to evaluate your working heart rate is the step test.

How to Determine Your Working Heart Rate: First, set up a sturdy box, stool, or other platform. You can also use a stair riser. It should be about 16 inches high. As briskly as you can, step onto and off the box. After 1 minute, stop and take your pulse for 15 seconds, then multiply the number by 4. That will give you your working heart rate. Divide that number by your max heart rate to determine the percentage of your max heart rate that you're working toward. Let's say you're age 33; your max heart rate is 187 (220 minus 33). If your poststepping pulse was 120, that's 64 percent of your max.

What Your Results Mean: Locate your score in the chart below to see where you stand. Everyone's working heart rate varies, and it's not uncommon for an individual's to go outside of the training zones shown below. Keep in mind, your working heart rate is only a gauge of fitness in relation to you as an individual and not to anyone else. Knowing this, you should closely monitor your heart rate throughout each workout, while continuing to push yourself as hard as you can.

Training Zones

AGE	BEATS PER MINUTE
25–29	140–170
30–34	136–169
35–39	132–160
40–44	128–155
45–49	117–150
50–54	115–145
55–59	113–140
60–64	111–135

Body Fat Distribution

TEST: Waist-to-Hip Ratio

The ratio of your waist-to-hip measurements is another good predictor of heart attack risk. One of the largest and most important cardiology studies ever conducted—the Interheart study—offers proof of this. From information on more than 27,000 people from 52 countries, researchers found that the higher a person's waist measurement relative to his hip measurement, the greater the risk of heart attack. Abdominal fat, say researchers, produces hormones and inflammatory substances that can be harmful to your heart and overall health. They published their results in the medical journal *The Lancet*.

How to Measure Your Waist-to-Hip Ratio: With a tape measure, stand in front of a mirror and measure your waist, which for the purposes of this test is the narrowest part of your midsection (this will usually be 2 to 3 inches above your navel). Divide that number by the circumference at your hip bones or at that point where your glutes protrude the most, whichever measurement is greater.

What Your Results Mean: The table below gives general guidelines for excellent to extreme levels for waist-to-hip ratio.

	EXCELLENT	GOOD	AVERAGE	HIGH	EXTREME
MALE	< 0.85	0.85–0.90	0.90–0.95	0.95–1.00	> 1.00
FEMALE	< 0.75	0.75–0.80	0.80–0.85	0.85–0.90	> 0.90

Flexibility

I'm big on flexibility. It's a key factor in becoming less vulnerable and more durable. Being flexible—and doing the work that builds flexibility—also increases strength. Flexibility seems to enhance the muscles' responsiveness, making them more receptive to strength stimuli like resistance training. A lack of flexibility, on the other hand, prevents each muscle from working through the most complete range of motion possible, which, if you work out, denies you all the benefits you're after in the first place.

Nowhere are strength and flexibility more important for me than on the ski slopes. With greater flexibility, especially in the hips, the knees are not asked to do something they are not designed for (namely, twist). When the snow gets heavy and crusty, normally a cause for tired groaning on my part, I feel strong, energized, and even coordinated, as long as my whole body is strong and flexible. The stronger and more flexible I am, the better I can ski to the bottom of a slope without my quads screaming in pain. I can even ski late into the day, without having to push through the drop-dead exhaustion that often hits other skiers. So prior to ski season, I always test my flexibility with the following exercises, and if needed, I amp up my flexibility work.

TEST: Hamstring Flexibility

This two-part test evaluates the range of motion in your hamstrings and your hip flexors. The less flexible this area is, the greater your chances of overstressing your lower back, making you prone to lower back pain and injury down the road.

How to Perform Part I of the Test: Lie flat on your back. Have a workout partner hold your left leg down with one hand and passively raise your right leg with the other hand. Make sure there's no pain in your lower back, along the glute, or deep inside the hamstring area, and do not bend your knee.

What Your Results Mean: For normal range of motion, your leg should raise to 80 to 85 degrees. Less than 80 degrees indicates tight hamstrings.

How to Perform Part 2 of the Test: Stay lying down on the floor, keeping your lower back flat. Grasp behind your left knee and pull your leg toward your chest.

What Your Results Mean: If your right leg stays flat to the floor, you have normal hip flexibility. If your right leg comes off the floor, this indicates shortened (tight) hip flexors. (Repeat with your right leg.)

TEST: Shoulder Flexibility

How to Perform the Test: Test your left shoulder by standing with your right arm straight up, then bend your elbow so your hand hangs behind your head. Keeping your upper arm stationary, rest your palm between your shoulder blades. Reach around behind you with your left arm so the palm is facing out, and try to touch the fingers of both hands together. Reverse the procedure and repeat with the opposite shoulder.

What Your Results Mean: Rate your flexibility according to the following:

   Good: Your fingers can touch.

   Fair: Your fingertips are not touching but are less than 2 inches apart.

   Poor: Your fingertips are more than 2 inches apart.

Muscular Strength and Endurance

TEST: Upper Body Strength

Upper body strength is important for a variety of sports, for injury prevention, and for daily activities like lifting children or carrying groceries.

How to Perform the Test: Find out how many modified pushups you can do without stopping. Begin by positioning your body correctly: Kneel on the floor. Keeping your weight on your knees, lean forward and place your palms flat on the floor about shoulder-width apart; your torso and thighs should be in a straight line. To do a pushup, lower your torso, keeping your back straight and abs tight, until your chest is about 3 inches above the floor. Then raise yourself back up to the starting position. Count the number of pushups you can complete in 1 minute.

What Your Results Mean: Below, find the number of pushups you did and rate your upper body strength accordingly:

> **Excellent:** 20 or more
>
> **Good:** 13 to 19
>
> **Fair:** 8 to 12
>
> **Poor:** Fewer than 8

TEST: Lower Body Strength

This test is designed to determine the muscular strength and endurance of your lower body. To perform this test you will need a chair (or equivalent) that allows you to squat with good form until your knees are bent at a 90-degree angle without actually sitting in the chair.

How to Perform the Test: Stand in front of a sturdy chair, feet hip-width apart. Cross your arms over your chest. Keeping your body weight over your heels, lower your torso as if you're going to sit on the chair seat. Stop just before your butt makes contact with the chair seat. Return to the standing position. That's one. Count the number you can do in 1 minute.

What Your Results Mean: Below, find the number of chair squats you did and rate your lower body strength accordingly.

> **Excellent:** 20 or more
>
> **Good:** 10 to 19
>
> **Fair:** 5 to 9
>
> **Poor:** 1 to 4

TEST: Core Strength

Core strength is important for everything from posture to sports performance to appearance. Plus, strong abs take stress off your lower back.

How to Perform the Test: See how many stomach crunches you can perform in 1 minute without stopping. To position your body the right way, lie on the floor with your knees bent and your feet flat on the floor. Place your palms facedown on your thighs. Lift your head and shoulders off the floor as you slide your hands up your legs until your fingertips touch your knees. To prevent neck strain, look up at the ceiling (not at your knees). Return to the starting position and repeat as many times as possible, counting as you go. If you need to hold your body in the starting position for more than a second, stop.

What Your Results Mean: Below, find the number of crunches you did and rate your core strength accordingly.

>   **Excellent:** 20 or more
>
>   **Good:** 10 to 19
>
>   **Fair:** 5 to 9
>
>   **Poor:** 1 to 4

Congratulations!

No matter what your scores are, don't feel discouraged. I've witnessed countless "miracle" turn-arounds in people, and I get emotional every time. Case in point: I have a very good friend whose name also happens to be Tony. He was very overweight (around 325 pounds), and, sadly, his condition triggered a heart attack. Can you imagine how scary that was for him and his wife, Dawn, who was also very out of shape? Tony and Dawn started rebuilding their health from poor to peak in every one of these evaluations. They kept at their workouts and changed their eating habits. They got healthy—so healthy, in fact, that Tony is now a certified fitness trainer and Dawn is a certified holistic health counselor. That's what I call a dramatic and dynamic 180-degree switch from who they were—and now they're helping others, to boot.

Next Steps

There's one evaluation tool I'd like you to de-emphasize: your bathroom scale. People let the scale tell them whether they're successful or not, especially when trying to lose weight. I tell my clients to stay away from the scale for a while. Focus instead on internal tools rather than external tools for gauging how you feel. Let your body give you regular reports on your progress. Are you less fatigued? Do you have more energy? Are you sleeping better? Do you feel stronger? Are your clothes getting looser? Most of the time, if you're eating what you're supposed to be eating and you're consistent with your workouts, you'll be answering "yes" to those questions.

I do think it's a good idea to take a picture of yourself before you start this program. Follow up by taking pictures every 4 weeks in the same outfit, whether it's a bathing suit or workout clothing, and then compare. You may not realize the changes your body is making on a daily basis, but the photographs can put things into perspective.

Your attitude is equally important. There's a fine line between a humble person, who works hard and is proud of his results, and someone who shouts his accomplishments from the rooftops. This "look at me" routine is part of the ego-fest that can jeopardize your long-term health and fitness, because it's based more on your need to be seen and less on your desire to be healthy. Turn off the act, be present in the moment, and listen to what's really happening. Stop looking for approval, and believe that your own health, fitness, and quality of life are far more important than how others perceive you.

Tony's Motivators: 7 Ways to a Perfect Day

I'm always looking for ways to enhance this amazing journey called life. For me, this often requires examining behavior where I've fallen short and trying to alter my approach the next time around. From this self-knowledge, I've created a list called The 7. When I do all 7, my day is as good as it gets.

1. **Sleep:** My perfect day starts the night before. If I get 7½ to 8 hours of sleep, I'm revved up and ready to hit the ground running. My body heals the best when I'm sleeping.

2. **Workout:** Like you didn't know this was going to be on the list! My workouts affect all aspects of my life—mind, body, spirit, and beyond. And while I exercise, I focus my thoughts on maximizing my workout.

3. **Whole foods:** Fruits, veggies, whole grains, lean protein, and healthy fats provide the fuel I need for a whole life.

4. **Supplements:** They assist with the recovery from workouts and provide energy for the next one.

5. **Attitude:** The more time spent asking questions to find solutions in life, the more exciting life becomes. Focus on what works, not on what doesn't.

6. **Charity:** Whether it's sending flowers to a friend, working with kids, or running in a race for charity, when you focus on others, you'll find true happiness. So choose something and sign up! Helping others who are less fortunate will make you feel grateful for the body you have.

7. **Downtime:** Turn off the tube. Read, meditate, or talk to people you love.

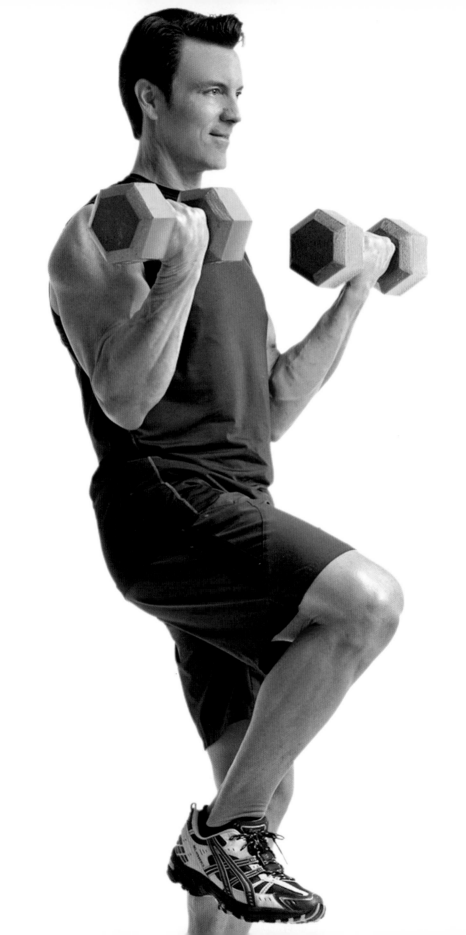

The Cycle of Success

Before we move into the actual exercises, workouts,

and nutrition plan, I want to make sure your head is in the right place. Many studies have shown that 50 percent of people who start an exercise program drop out within 6 months. Afterward, they feel stuck and disheartened. Can you relate? These feelings trigger a negative cycle of self-doubt and decreased levels of motivation and performance, resulting in a downward health spiral.

It takes more than physical stamina to stick with a training program. Researchers are finding that people who change their health and lifestyle for the better don't just alter the way they eat and exercise. They condition their mental skills, too.

I want to help you do that with my motivational system: the Cycle of Success. What makes the Cycle of Success so powerful is that in successive turns of the wheel, it creates internal motivation. People with internal motivation exercise for intrinsic reasons (interest, enjoyment, and challenge), and their adherence rates are much higher. People who are internally motivated tend to spend time on exercise because it brings individual emotional satisfaction. Those who are externally motivated by improving their appearance are generally less devoted.

Apply each turn of the wheel in the Cycle of Success, and you'll learn to treat yourself well (with kindness, self-acceptance, tolerance, and no criticism). Your self-confidence will improve. Your attitude will brighten. Flowers will spontaneously bloom in your presence. You'll appreciate your body more and realize that great health is the foundation of success in every endeavor. And your life will look better all around. All of this results in a positive, self-perpetuating cycle of success with amazing forward momentum. Here's how the Cycle of Success works—and how it will work for you.

Ask for What You Need

Do you need more time to exercise? How about some help with a particular exercise technique? Is your family giving you enough support in your fitness efforts?

If not, ask for what you need (whatever it is). Reluctance to reach out is all too common in our culture, where self-reliance is a revered, ingrained habit. Asking for help often feels like a personal failure. We think we look stupid if it appears we don't have all the answers. Asking for assistance—such as for help managing your household or workload, a deadline extension, or even feedback—doesn't signal incompetence. On the contrary, though you may feel vulnerable, what you're really saying is "I want to do this right, and I understand the value of support and cooperation."

Turning to others in times of need is also a sign of strength and smarts because it means you know what you can and can't handle and that you're planning ahead to get things done, regardless.

A very close friend and business colleague of mine, Traci Morrow, is a wife and mom with six children. That family profile alone might make you think she has very little time to exercise. Wrong. Traci is a 6-days-a-week exerciser who is in superb shape. She has mastered this part of the cycle; she asks for what she needs.

"Long ago, I realized I'd need to reconsider my attitude about asking for help if I wanted things to run smoothly, especially after we became a family of eight," Traci told me. She doesn't hesitate to request the assistance she needs, either, whether it's sending her husband grocery shopping, tapping her daughter to do chores, or asking a neighbor to babysit her kids while she goes to the gym. The result: She's calm, confident, and supremely focused.

And Traci is motivated by the positive impact her requests have had. "My kids are learning responsibility and benefiting from a feeling of accomplishment when they do small chores. I had to learn to ask for help, but now I can't imagine living my life any other way."

Ask for what you need. I do it all the time because I am not an expert by any means. Everything I say and everything I do is a collection of all the questions that I have asked over the years.

Here's an example from my life: A few years ago, I developed a piece of exercise equipment called PowerStands. It helps people put more depth into their pushups, without having to place their hands on hard surfaces or straining their wrists. I called three people to find out who could make a prototype. I asked for what I needed: Who could do it within my budget? Who could make it with the right materials, in terms of durability, stability, and weight? Should I patent it or trademark it? By asking for what I needed, I was able to develop my PowerStands pushup equipment and bring it to market successfully. There is no way that would have happened had I not kept making phone calls and asking knowledgeable people for advice.

Who are the people that you rely on to find the answers you need? Are you okay with the fact that maybe the first, second, or third source you go to may not be able to give you all of the answers?

Anytime you ask someone for a significant favor, be clear and succinct about what you want. Boil down the main idea into a few sentences so that your point can be easily understood. Don't talk in long, complicated paragraphs and examples. If necessary, acknowledge that your request is a big deal ("I know I'm asking a lot"), and give the person you are asking permission to decline up front ("I'll understand if it's too much and you can't do it").

When you ask for information, listen closely and consider the answers. Carefully process what you hear. Has this person's advice worked for other people? Take the good advice. Leave the bad advice. Then proceed based on the best wisdom you've gathered.

Don't Get Fooled Again

I can't emphasize this enough, or in too many ways: If it sounds too good to be true, it's probably not worth your time or your dime. Stay away from programs that promise unrealistic results; promote the idea of superfast weight loss; require you to purchase special products, supplements, or foods; or include claims that a certain elixir wipes out diseases. Don't fall victim to claims of extreme weight loss from actors, models, or other celebrities who endorse dangerous diets and pieces of exercise equipment. If it were that easy to lose weight, everyone would be slim and trim. That's not happening. Americans are getting fatter. Experts suggest that 75 percent of Americans will be overweight by 2015, and 41 percent of that group will be obese. By the time many of us realize that fads and gimmicks are no substitute for good eating habits and a sensible exercise program, we will have paid a very expensive price.

The honest-to-God truth is that weight is managed by diet and exercise. The underlying principle is simple in theory and can be summarized by the phrase "energy balance." Energy balance is the difference between *energy in* (calories consumed in diet) and *energy out* (calories burned through physical activity). All things held constant, regularly consuming more calories than you burn leads to a positive energy balance that packs on pounds. Conversely, eat fewer calories than you burn, and you'll experience a negative energy balance and fat loss.

So whatever you're doing, if it's not working, then stop doing it. Don't be fooled again.

Do Scary Things That Don't Kill You

Do you avoid the gym because you're afraid you'll reveal to the world that you're uncoordinated and out of shape? Do you want to get physically fit, but the thought of trying something new intimidates you? Are you afraid of making a fool of yourself or looking silly?

If you've been dreaming of doing more with your life both in the gym and outside of it, let this book be your catalyst for change. What's holding you back? Fear? Lack of confidence? Procrastination? Lack of purpose? In the long run, it's better to face your fears, or as I say, "Do scary things that don't kill you." Facing your fears is the best way to conquer them.

Fifteen years ago, I signed up for my very first extreme ski camp in Red Mountain, a little-known behemoth of a ski area in southern British Columbia, just across the border from Washington State. To get there, I had to fly into Portland, Oregon, rent a car, and navigate my way to the Canadian border where surly looking guards scrutinized my passport and searched my rental car.

I finally pulled up to the resort in the early evening. Every run looked like a cliff: treacherous, with ragged ridges and near-vertical drops. The classic definition of extreme skiing popped into my head: You fall, you die. Red Mountain is the kind of place where, if you make a wrong turn, the ski patroller finds your body—in June. I was scared, really scared.

So there I was by myself, but with a bunch of strangers at this extreme ski camp. That night at dinner, I listened to their stories about Red Mountain. There's a lot of through-the-trees skiing, they said. There's white-knuckle terrain . . . a 1,400-foot vertical drop . . . willingness to test your limits . . . avalanche potential . . . cliff jumping for the particularly adventurous. I began thinking this camp was the worst idea I'd ever had in my life. I had nightmares about spending my days hurtling off cliffs with kick-ass skiers.

My mission: to get home in one piece.

The next morning, I found out pretty quickly that we would not be eased into this experience. We were sent to the top of the mountain, and everyone dispersed. As I stood there facing the woods, alone, I had not only forgotten everything I ever knew about skiing, I was sure I had forgotten everything that anybody ever knew about skiing.

Then I let out a yell that sounded like a cross between a war whoop and a death rattle, and I took off. I cranked one turn, and then another, and another.

At noon, I sat down with some of the other guys. I expressed how thrilled I was to have survived long enough to have lunch.

Over the course of the 4 days, a strange thing happened. My fears all but disappeared. My skiing improved markedly, but it was really an attitude adjustment that had me doing runs on terrain

I once thought reserved for mountain goats. By the end of the camp, I realized it was the greatest thing I had ever done.

The experience wasn't about hurtling myself off a 150-foot cliff. It was about facing my fears—and being able to look back up at the hill and say to myself, "Hey, I skied that." I signed up for another extreme ski camp. To date, I've attended more than 14 of these terrifying camps—and enjoyed every one.

People who come to my fitness classes have the same fears and apprehensions I did when going to my first extreme ski camp. They are scared to death. They're afraid of collapsing in the middle of one of my workouts, in front of everyone.

But without risk, there's little reward. What is one goal that fear has kept you from pursuing? Face your fears by taking a step toward your goals today.

Find Your Mentor(s)

There is a way to get what you want in a shorter period of time: Find a successful mentor who has already achieved what you want. Success leaves a trail of (whole wheat) bread crumbs. When people are successful at something, whether they have a great relationship, are extraordinarily successful in business, or have the body that you desire, it's not because they won the lottery. It's because they applied a set of strategies, and those strategies work. You don't need to reinvent the wheel to find a way to succeed. Throughout my life, I've always believed it's been best to learn from successful people.

Seek out a mentor whom you respect and whose advice you want. A mentor doesn't have to be an authority, just someone who has achieved the success you're after. Most people are flattered to be asked to be a mentor and feel an immediate sense of pride.

When asking for help, tell your mentor your main challenge and the actions you've taken thus far. Avoid asking for too much information; rather, ask a question that can be answered in a few minutes. Don't ask "How do I develop a fitter body?" Instead, simply ask "What are three actions I can take right now to get in better shape?" Learn from his or her wisdom; then walk the talk.

Be a mentor yourself. When you give people an opportunity to be independent, confident, and exposed to new ideas, you don't just have an impact, you help them transform their lives. A few years ago, I attended my 30th high school reunion. I ended up hanging out with a classmate named Ann and her fiancé, Bob. In high school, Ann was a perfect size 2, a cheerleader, and one of the cool chicks who wouldn't design to talk to me. She had put on weight over the years, eventually growing to a size 16, a fact she covered up at the reunion by wearing baggy black clothes. Naturally, the conversation drifted to fitness and working out and ended with the three of us making plans to ski together at Crested Butte. (Yes, I am about to tell another ski story!)

Fast-forward to our ski trip: Ann told me that she couldn't believe that I was skiing harder and faster than the younger people there (I was 49 at the time). "You are fitter, you are faster, you are stronger than you were 31 years ago!" she said.

Then came the big question: Ann wanted to know how she could lose weight, get fit, ski better, and have more fun in life.

I got her started on P90X and asked her to commit to it 100 percent for the full 90 days. "Your only job is to show up and pay attention to what happens when you get there," I told her.

Ann agreed to my terms. I checked in with her weekly to see how she was doing and to help her take her workouts up a notch.

Ann gave the program 110 percent and more. She shrank to a size 6 and now looks fabulous. Her whole life changed. Today she's a fitness coach, loving her life and doing extremely well financially.

You never know what believing in someone or being kind will do for them. You may never realize the true influence your support has on another. But if you are steadfast in your faith in them, miracles can happen.

Think and Act Outside the Box

Don't be afraid to be a pioneer in your own life about the things you need. Be innovative and think and act outside the box. Another personal story: Many of the workouts I design include plyometrics (jump training). I realize that's a new concept for many people, so I used to give exercisers the usual in-the-box advice: Before they can do plyometrics, they need a good surface, sturdy shoes, and an understanding of how to modify the exercises. Then I started thinking outside the box: Why don't I invent something that makes plyometrics even easier on the body—something that eases the landing and helps you launch, as gymnasts do on their special flooring?

So I got to work on designing a portable gymnastics floor. It turns plyometrics into a training system that most people can do, even if they have some physical limitations.

Think outside the box by trying some new foods and recipes (start with the ones in this book!), working with a nutritionist, or making a commitment to learn my exercises. Also, you have to think outside the box after you've progressed to the Warrior level and completed 6 weeks of Warrior level training. What should you do then? Get creative. Mix your workouts in with bike riding, salsa classes, kickboxing, parkour—whatever suits you. Revisit your Fitness Quotient for new ideas. I've seen hundreds of people come up with creative, innovative ways to stay in the game, prevent boredom, and combat the plateau effect.

Do Nothing

I know you're saying, "Whaaaaat . . . you want me to stop and do nothing?" That's right—for 15 minutes each day, do nothing. Sit in the quietness. Center yourself before taking on the challenges of the day. Visualize the new body you're creating, or prop yourself up in a chair and just breathe—no TV, laptop, or cell phone. Try meditation, quiet time, prayer, or anything that helps you hear the truth and the deeper voice that will help you lead the proper life. When it's warm and sunny, I go out to my backyard and sit in the sun. I'm not wasting time, either; I'm doing myself a lot of good. Just 10 to 15 minutes of sunshine helps the body synthesize vitamin D. By "doing nothing," I'm doing something: fortifying myself with a much-needed vitamin and enjoying therapeutic downtime. There's more: I get some of my most creative thoughts and solutions during my downtime. I'm thus a true believer in doing nothing. It keeps me in a peaceful, creative place.

Why is doing nothing of so much value? In two words, *yin* and *yang*. Yin and yang represent the Chinese understanding of energy flow through the body. Yang is active and yin is restful. The two forces are opposite, yet mutually supportive, and in constant flux. When there are equal amounts of both forces, body, mind, and spirit are in harmony. But usually, they're out of balance. Our modern lifestyles generate many sources of stress, poor nutrition, and insufficient exercise; in addition, our bodies are exposed to harsh climates and pollution. The hectic pace we set for our lives builds up an almost unbearable pressure (too much yang) and creates a kind of pain within us that is difficult to heal without a real commitment to living differently. All of this disturbs the natural flow of energy throughout the body. Balance can be restored in a variety of ways, including through diet and exercise, as well as through personal quiet time (doing nothing), which relaxes the body and mind to improve the flow of energy.

Carve out a part of your day to do nothing. It probably shouldn't be right after you get out of bed; it's usually too tough to focus. After breakfast, before lunch, before you go to bed at night—find the best time for you. In the nothingness, you'll learn more about yourself, what you need to do about who you are becoming, and what is important in your life. True success in life—and in health and fitness—comes when there is balance, Grasshopper.

Finish What You Start

Ever have one of those days when you decide to quit smoking, start exercising, or dedicate yourself to something like finishing a marathon? Anthony has. But before that day, all he would do after work was smoke pot and lie on the couch, stuffing himself with fast-food tacos. His weight shot up to 240 pounds.

"Finally, I just put a stake in the ground and said, 'I'm done,'" he said in a letter to me. Anthony started doing P90X. He stuck with it, following it to the letter. The lessons he learned from sticking to that workout translated into his personal life. The smoking and the excess weight became things of the past.

"Sometimes you want to quit, but then you finish it. Completion is a dimension of being successful. Training with goals in mind opens up a world of possibilities. Now I'm very into accomplishing big things," he says. Getting in shape had a cascading effect on Anthony's life. He's now studying to be a fitness trainer.

Lesson: Don't jump from one thing to another, leaving a string of unfinished chores or goals behind you. Finish what you start because your past efforts will pay off. I used to be a procrastinator until I realized that I had to finish things to be successful. Now, every time I see something through to the very end, I experience success, whether it's completing the prototype for a new invention or learning a new skill like rock climbing. I've discovered that perseverance is a character trait worth developing and procrastination is a trait to ditch.

Do what I do: Write the word "FINISH" with a bright red magic marker at the top of your calendar. It will help you make that call, write that e-mail, finish that project, or complete your workouts. I look at that word, and it motivates me to follow through. Also, make a list of things that bother you and need to be completed, repaired, or finalized. My list includes things like hanging new curtains in my bedroom, letting go of a grudge, and painting my deck. Then finish the things on your list, one by one.

And speaking of following through, complete the workouts and nutrition plan in this book. Follow the steps to becoming a Warrior; stick to the nutrition plan for 30 days. Can you do it? Yes! Start small, think big, work hard, finish what you start, and never quit. Not to boast, but personally I'm careful never to leave anything unfini—

Have a Hobby

What does a hobby have to do with health, fitness, and wellness? Everything! A hobby can transport you away from your daily troubles and stress or keep you from indulging in destructive habits. I've also read that hobbies, if they're interesting and stimulating, can help preserve your mental vitality by challenging your brain. When choosing a hobby, find one that uses as many senses as possible, such as sculpting, painting, or learning a new language. And make sure it's something you enjoy.

One of my hobbies is coin collecting. I'm always fishing through change and bills. There's history in my hand. If I find a quarter from 1954—before I was born—I start wondering: What was going on in the world then? Whose hands held this quarter? Coin collecting is important to me because it's a stress-relieving activity that gets me out of my normal routine. It gives me great joy. It calms me down quite a bit. I think it makes me a better person.

For a lot of people I've met, fitness has become their hobby. And for many of them, what started out as a hobby has become a career in fitness—as coaches, personal trainers, fitness instructors, and nutritionists.

Choose Right over Wrong

We all have to make choices and be accountable for the consequences. Our responsibility is to define our priorities, weigh the consequences, and choose right over wrong. Let's say you think you don't have time to exercise. So you don't. You avoid considering the eventual consequences of your couch-potato lifestyle, as if by magic those consequences might not one day visit you personally. Stroke, heart attack, diabetes? Not me, please. In general, people like to shrug off personal responsibility for their actions, particularly if those actions have negative consequences. The truth is, wrong choices eventually lead to chaos.

How can you make better choices? Using the example above again, evaluate how you're currently using your time and explore what changes can be made. Let's say that while you leave for work by 8:15 a.m., you don't get up until 7:30. Find extra time to exercise by getting up an hour earlier. Look at your present schedule and determine how you can rearrange it to accommodate an exercise routine.

Our choices should typically be guided by what's right, not necessarily by what's easiest, most comfortable, or most convenient. That's really what self-discipline is all about. A healthy lifestyle teaches us that.

So ask yourself: Do you want benefits or do you want negative consequences? It's you who gets to choose. The exciting news is that the personal responsibility you develop through a fit, active lifestyle will transfer to the rest of your life as you begin to take control of all that you do.

Remember: Choose wrong and here come the problems, sooner or later. Life is not about instant gratification. One of my mantras early on was "Short-term pain and discomfort can lead to a lifetime of excitement, wellness, happiness, and joy. Short-term pleasure can lead to a myriad of problems." That is a universal truth, and you can hang your hat on it.

Do What You Love, Love What You Do . . .

And the money will come. While I was growing up, the biggest issue in our home was money. My mother and dad, when they argued, it was always about money—how much he made, how it was invested, what they spent, how to pay the bills, and on and on. It was a constant battle, and it was stressful to me as a little kid. I didn't want my parents' beliefs about money to be my beliefs, so over the years I've created new beliefs that are more closely aligned with my goals and values.

A common misconception is that money—and plenty of it—is the key to a happy life. Sure, in order to be happy we do need the basics (it's rough to be cheery when you are sitting in the rain because you don't have a roof over your head while your tummy screams at you for some food), but after our basic needs are met, it seems that money contributes little to our level of happiness. It is true: Money doesn't buy happiness. Okay—so what does?

I believe that when we're engaged in the right activity, we experience a state of mind referred to as "flow," in which we're completely engrossed in the experience and feel truly alive. Talk to anyone who has spent a big portion of their time engaged or absorbed in a specific activity, and you'll find a happier person than someone who has lived a less-engaged existence.

Spend as much time as you can in a state of flow to achieve happiness. This could be a hobby, a sport, a workout, or all of the above. Achieving flow at work is critical, too; after all, we do spend almost half of our waking life at work. Do what you love! If your job is a grind and you don't know what you love to do, think back to what you loved to do as a kid. When I was a child, I loved being silly and making people laugh. I eventually used my sense of humor to help me become a stand-up comic and a TV personality. Even today, as a trainer, my sense of humor guides the way I interact with clients and help people get fit. I try to make people laugh, have fun, and enjoy life.

Getting laughs helped me get by when I was young, but my brain and my heart were telling me that there was more to life. In my twenties, I had the wherewithal to seek betterment for myself. Which brings me to the other "secret" to happiness: the need to know that your life has significance, that it has meaning. From what is meaning derived? It starts with a conviction that we are of value and have something worthwhile to contribute. It is fostered by knowing that we are a part of something bigger than ourselves and, like an organ of the body, are necessary and needed.

Find the Funny

We all have the power to choose our reaction to a difficult situation: We can overreact, get angry (even at ourselves), and risk making things even worse—or we can just lighten up.

Imagine calling your doctor and hearing him say, "Watch two comedy movies and call me in the morning." Laughter is a great healer. Studies show it lowers blood pressure, reduces stress hormones, increases muscle flexion, and boosts immune function by raising levels of T cells, which fight infection, and B cells, which produce disease-destroying antibodies. Laughter also triggers the release of endorphins, the body's natural painkillers, and produces an overall sense of well-being.

Have you ever watched children at play and noticed how easily and heartily they laugh? We should all be like that. Ben Franklin once wrote, "Some people die at 25 but aren't buried until they're 75." Laughter and humor teach us how to live! Why not allow their healing powers to improve your health and happiness?

Lighten up. Don't give yourself such a hard time. You don't have to be perfect like me. (See—that's me being funny.) A sense of humor opens doors, releases tension, and builds new friendships and business opportunities. Run from gloom and doom, and surround yourself with happy, shiny people.

Finally, keep in mind that the first three letters of *funny* are f-u-n. Fun and funny go together. When you're laughing, you're having fun (but you probably knew that already).

Be Amazing

Imagine if every day you woke up and said the following mantra: "I am going to be amazing today." How would such an affirmation guide your days?

To be amazing, you have to first be authentic. You may not be aware that there are two versions of you. You have a "real self," whom you were created to be, and a "fictional self," whom the world has told you to be.

If you're like most people, you're living your fictional self. You may have spent the greater part of your life worrying about what other people think of you and spending most of your energy in an effort to please them. You must stop caring about what other people think. A strong need to be liked and admired can make someone extremely sensitive to criticism. Rather than focus on what people think, celebrate your victories and accomplishments and recognize the things you do really well.

What makes most people go crazy is thinking they have to live up to their reputation. But your reputation is not the result of what you think about you—it's based on what other people think. Are you driven by what somebody else believes you to be? You are not your reputation. You are not what other people think of you. You are what *you* think of you!

Your real self is not defined by what others think, nor by the roles (wife/husband, mom/dad, employee/boss) you have in life. It is defined by the genuine substance of who you are at your very core. It's the sum of your thoughts, talents, wisdom, and skills. It's that which makes you, amazingly, you.

When you're not living as your real self, you probably wake up each day with an inner gnawing, a hunger for more, the feeling that something is missing in your life. You may find yourself feeling incomplete, anxious, confused, and overwhelmed. In other words, not amazing.

Being amazing is a lifelong pursuit. If you aren't living a 100 percent amazing life today, you're not alone—most of us aren't! Recognize the things you can do to make your life more amazing, and do one thing each day to improve your life.

Bring It!

Before you get moving with the routines in Part 2, let's sum things up. To start out on the right path, live in the Cycle of Success. Ask for help, don't fall for gimmicks, stand up for what you believe, face your fears, find mentors, and be creative. Practice clearing your mind, observing your thoughts, and discrediting those that don't serve you. Finish what you start. Engage yourself in a hobby or two. Choose right over wrong. Lighten up. Do what you love, love what you do.

The same opportunity for change can happen in your personal life if you make health and fitness your priority now. If you feel miserable, tired, and self-conscious, how can you possibly be the amazing person that awaits you?

Do you have limits? Who has set them—you or someone else? You are best able to decide what you can do, where you can go, and how high you can climb. Once you realize this, your life will become more rewarding—and fun, as well!

A personal renaissance is waiting in your head at the intersection of "I can't" and "I can."

Which path will you take?

PART 2 The Routines

Now that you've diagnosed your fitness level and capacity and know where to start, it's time to . . . well, start! In Part 2, you'll find the routine that fits you: Beginner, Striver, or Warrior. For each fitness level, you'll find a list of the exercises designed for you and your suggested weekly schedule. Read through all of this—and get excited!

One of the reasons why these routines will work for you—especially if you've tried and failed with other programs—is that they do not draw from one form of exercise. They incorporate a variety of things: strength building, plyometrics, abdominal and core work, boxing and kickboxing, yoga, stretching, and cardiovascular exercises. I've always tried to make my routines fun and filled with a variety of movements. They're uncomplicated, easy to follow, and time-tested, with combinations that work. These routines are the "on switch" to a lifetime of health and fitness.

Have fun with your new fitness plan, and don't freak out if you don't see results in the first 45 days. "What?! No results in the first month and a half?!" See, I knew you'd freak out. The reality is that we all have different starting points. Some of you will see results within a week—lucky you! Others of you might have to wait a little longer, based on your age, body weight, fitness level, flexibility, balance, athletic background, and so on. This is normal. The variety of moves purposely plays into your strengths and weaknesses. Be patient. Your body will adapt, and you will be amazed at how you look and feel.

Once you've familiarized yourself with your routine, keep reading. The exercise instructions will follow in Part 3. Stay with it—and stay positive!

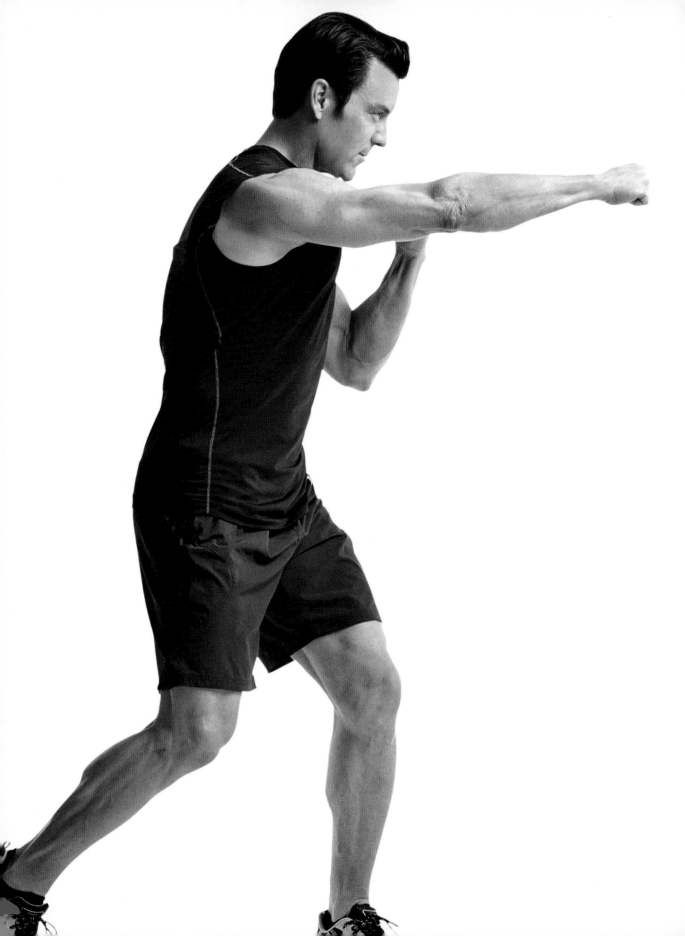

5

The Beginner's Workout

If the results of my Fitness Quotient test indicate that you're a Beginner, this might mean you haven't been a fan of exercise in the past. Perhaps you're intimidated by the gym or you don't enjoy working out. Or maybe you have a physical condition that has temporarily sidelined you. Don't worry—I'm going to ease you into an exercise routine that is custom-made for you. And in just a few short weeks, you will begin to look better, feel better, and change your life.

What You Need to Get Started

You don't need a lot of equipment to get a great workout at home. For a relatively minimal investment—much cheaper than an annual gym membership—you can get everything you need. For the exercises in this book, you will need:

Resistance bands. These are available in a variety of resistance levels: light, medium, and heavy resistance (usually color-coded yellow, green, and red). Purchase two different colors to have on hand during workouts.

Exercise bench. Sometimes the floor just doesn't cut it, and your carpeting might irritate your skin. Invest in a simple adjustable bench. It can be used for many exercises, and on certain moves it allows you to go through a greater range of motion than the floor does.

Exercise mat. Purchase a lightweight mat that rolls up easily and provides support and comfort for floor exercises like pushups, crunches, and stretches. Mats also help cushion your knees and back.

Space. A dedicated space is great, but any open area will do. Add a CD player or radio for melodic motivation, a towel to wipe those beads of sweat, and, if possible, a mirror in which to check your form—and your results!

A Two-Phase Plan

Each workout in this book includes two phases. For Beginners, both phases are approximately 20 minutes long and thus easy to squeeze into your schedule. Phase 1 is designed to get your body acclimated to exercise and help you learn my basic style of training. I suggest you do Beginner's Phase 1 for 3 weeks, then advance to Beginner's Phase 2. In Phase 2, the intensity of your workout increases. Stay on Phase 2 for 3 weeks. These two phases will help you build a solid foundation for developing lean muscle, flexibility, and cardiovascular conditioning.

Because your muscles respond more positively to continued stresses, you need to give them a sustained growth stimulus. So after 6 weeks at the Beginner level, you're ready to move on to the Striver level. The end result will be adaptation—the exercise scientist's fancy word for progress. And progress is what it's all about.

The Circuit Solution

My cardio and resistance training workouts are organized in "circuits." Circuit training is a workout technique in which you move from one exercise to another, one set per movement per round, with minimal rest in between. You'll be on the move constantly during these workouts. The continuous nature of circuit training keeps your metabolism high throughout the workout.

Circuits are a superior way to train. In fact, a very recent study from the University of Padua in Italy supports this point. Researchers assigned 40 people (ages 50 to 65) to a control group or to one of three exercise groups: an endurance group, a strength-training group, and a circuit-training group. At the end of the experimental period (12 weeks), those who did circuit training lost the most fat (particularly around the waist) and the most overall weight. Plus, they made more strength gains than the other groups.[1] Circuit training is the best way to get results.

Your Caloric Burn

I asked fitness coach Mark Briggs, one of my associates, to do an independent test of each workout in this book in order to calculate caloric burn. According to Mark's evaluation, the Beginner's workout burns 200 to 300 calories—and that's in just 20 minutes! Keep in mind that there are several variables when it comes to calories burned. Your age, weight, conditioning, workout intensity, and speed of movement are all factors that address how many calories you burn in a specified workout. Once you get familiar with the exercises and the workout and can increase your level of intensity, your caloric burn rate will move to the upper end of the range. When that happens, you can potentially burn a little more than a half pound a week, if you work out 6 days a week for 20 minutes each time. Here's why: There are 3,500 calories in 1 pound of fat. If you do the Beginner's workout for 6 days and burn 300 calories each time, that adds up to a calorie deficit of 1,800 calories, which is a little more than a half pound.

Getting Results

Begin any workout program and the first thing on your mind is going to be how long you have to wait before you see results. Most Beginners make fantastic gains in strength, tone, and stamina during their first few weeks. If you're dedicated and consistent, these benefits will come. The following guidelines will help you continue on your path to success.

Familiarize yourself with the exercise movements before doing a complete routine. Carefully study the exercise descriptions and photos and do a practice run-through to familiarize yourself with the movements; then concentrate on performing the exercises correctly. Once your body is accustomed to the movements, you can begin to perform the exercises back-to-back with some momentum.

Be conscious of your form. Keep every muscle tight as you progress through each repetition. Hold your abs and your glutes tight always. Allow your lower back to keep its natural arch, and maintain good posture with your shoulders down and chest forward. For standing movements, keep a slight bend in your knees.

Perform only those exercises that appear in the routines for your fitness level. If a specific exercise is giving you a lot of trouble or doesn't feel right, try one of my modifications.

Do the exact number of repetitions listed for each exercise. You can continue to add more resistance (i.e., a heavier-resistance band) to exercises that feel easy, provided that the additional load doesn't cause you to lose proper form. Remember, performing any exercise properly is more important than adding extra weight or resistance.

Where indicated, shoot for "max reps." This refers to the point in an exercise set at which you can't complete another rep without breaking your form. In most instances, your form starts to deteriorate before you realize it, and you begin to incorporate secondary muscles into the movement instead of using strictly the targeted muscles.

When you rest, do so briefly. If you have time to chat on your cell phone during your workout, don't plan on losing fat. You must keep rest periods between sets to a minimum. Research shows that resistance workouts that incorporate short rest periods not only challenge your body more during the workout itself but also lead to a much more dramatic spike in the production of fat-burning hormones afterward. I believe in rest intervals of no longer than 30 seconds. (It's a good idea to wear a watch with a second hand to monitor rest intervals.) Learning how to manipulate your rest intervals between sets can turn an ordinary workout into an extraordinary one.

Focus on the task at hand. As you get into your workout, ignite a ferocious flame of training energy and zeal. Keep distractions to a minimum (put the dog outside, turn off the TV, drop the kids off at a friend's house) so that you can really concentrate on your workout and get into the "zone." A favorite music selection can help you get cranked up, too.

Follow my suggested training schedule (see page 58) and plan your week accordingly.

Beginner's Cardio Phase I

The Warmup
Your warmup consists of a brief cardiovascular workout (General Warmup) and stretching (Specific Warmup). The General Warmup warms up your muscles and joints, preparing you for your workout.

The Specific Warmups include light stretches to limber up your muscles and connective tissues (ligaments, tendons) for the work to follow. Carefully and slowly stretch a tight muscle until it reaches its normal degree of suppleness. Skipping either the General or Specific Warmup will increase the likelihood of injury and make you less able to use more resistance in the exercises. Err on the side of caution—you're always better off doing too much warmup work than too little!

General Warmup

Walk in place (20 steps)

Jog in place (30 steps)

Run in place (40 steps)

Walk in place (20 steps)

Specific Warmup

Side Stretch

Yoga Hamstring Stretch

Runner's Stretch

Standing Quad Stretch

The Workout (20 reps per move)

Circuit 1

Step Jacks

Line Leaps

Jab/Cross

Squat Walk

30-second rest, then repeat Circuit 1

30-second rest after repeating Circuit 1, then move to Circuit 2

Circuit 2

Pivot Punches

Lateral Shuffle, with arms up

Front Kicks

30-second rest, then move to the Cooldown

Cooldown

To wind down your body, aid recovery, and reduce postexercise muscular soreness, cool down after your workout is complete. This will help your heart, lungs, and blood flow return to their normal state. If you abruptly stop moving, blood pools in the muscles you were using, which can cause dizziness and fainting.

Spend 5 to 10 minutes on the following series of progressive stretches to cover all your major muscle groups.

March in place to bring down your heart rate (20 steps).

Side Stretch

Yoga Hamstring Stretch

Runner's Stretch

Standing Quad Stretch

Beginner's Cardio Phase 2

General Warmup

Walk in place (20 steps)

Jog in place (30 steps)

Run in place (40 steps)

Jog in place (30 steps)

Specific Warmup

Side Stretch

Yoga Hamstring Stretch

Runner's Stretch

Standing Quad Stretch

The Workout (20 reps per move)

Circuit I

Step Jacks

Line Leaps

Jab/Cross

Squat Walk

30-second rest, then repeat Circuit I

30-second rest after repeating Circuit I, then move to Circuit 2

Circuit 2

Pivot Punches

Lateral Shuffle, with arms up

Front Kicks

30-second rest and repeat Circuit 2, then move to the Cooldown

Cooldown

March in place to bring down your heart rate (20 steps).

Side Stretch

Yoga Hamstring Stretch

Runner's Stretch

Standing Quad Stretch

Beginner's Resistance Phase I

General Warmup

Walk in place (20 steps)

Jog in place (30 steps)

Run in place (40 steps)

Specific Warmup

Head Rolls

Shoulder Rolls

Side Stretch

Arm Circles

Huggers

Yoga Hamstring Stretch, with feet wide apart

Yoga Hamstring Stretch

Downward-Facing Dog

The Workout

Circuit 1

Standard Pushups, or from knees for Modified Pushups (max reps)

Standing Shoulder Presses, with dumbbells (15–20 reps)

Standing Biceps Curls (10–15 reps)

Standing Double-Arm Triceps Presses (10–15 reps)

Shoulder-Width Squats (20–30 reps)

Crunches (max reps)

30-second rest, then repeat Circuit 1

30-second rest after repeating Circuit 1, then move to Circuit 2

Circuit 2

Wide-Hand Pushups (max reps)

Upright Rows, with dumbbells (10–15 reps)

21s

Wide-Feet Squats (20–30 reps)

In and Out Crunches (max reps)

30-second rest, then move to the Cooldown

Cooldown

Shoulder Rolls (alternate 8 to the left, 8 to the right)

Double Backstroke (8 reps)

Double Front Stroke (8 reps)

Huggers

Yoga Hamstring Stretch, with feet wide apart

Yoga Hamstring Stretch

Downward-Facing Dog

Beginner's Resistance Phase 2

General Warmup

Walk in place (20 steps)

Jog in place (30 steps)

Run in place (40 steps)

Jog in place (30 steps)

Specific Warmup

Head Rolls

Shoulder Rolls

Double Backstroke (8 reps)

Double Front Stroke (8 reps)

Huggers

Yoga Hamstring Stretch, with feet wide apart

Yoga Hamstring Stretch

Downward-Facing Dog

Standing Quad Stretch

The Workout

Circuit I

Standard Pushups, or from knees for Modified Pushups (max reps)

Lawnmowers (10–15 reps on each side)

Standing Shoulder Presses (15–20 reps)

Standing Biceps Curls (10–15 reps)

Standing Double-Arm Triceps Presses (10–15 reps)

Shoulder-Width Squats (20–30 reps)

Crunches (max reps)

30-second rest, then repeat Circuit I

30-second rest after repeating Circuit I, then move to Circuit 2

Circuit 2

Wide-Hand Pushups (max reps)

Bent-Over Rows (10–15 reps)

Upright Rows, with dumbbells (10–15 reps)

21s

Wide-Feet Squats (20–30 reps)

In and Out Crunches (30–50 reps)

30-second rest, then move to the Cooldown

Special Age-Related Advice for Beginners

Congratulations on getting into the game, or back into the game. It's important to take the right precautions to help you make the most of your experience. If you have not been exercising regularly, please have a medical examination, unless you are under age 30 and have had a satisfactory checkup within the past year. If you are over 30 . . .

30 to 34 years: Have a medical examination that includes a resting electrocardiograph (EKG).

35 to 44 years: Have a medical exam and preexercise testing, including an exercise stress test. A physician can identify any contraindications to exercise as your response to increasingly difficult levels of work is monitored on an EKG.

45 to 64 years: Have a full medical examination, plus a stress test. If you have any health concerns, consult your doctor about preexisting conditions before you begin an exercise program.

65 years and older: The same advice holds here: a complete medical examination, stress test, and evaluation of preexisting medical conditions to look for signs of complications. Your doctor may advise against certain exercises, such as higher-impact moves if you have joint problems or foot problems due to diabetes.

Regardless of your age, consult your doctor if you have two or more of the following risk factors: high blood pressure, high cholesterol, or diabetes, or if you are a smoker or have a family history of early onset heart disease (first-degree relative with heart disease before age 65 for female relatives, or before age 55 for male relatives).

Cooldown

Shoulder Rolls

Double Backstroke (8 reps)

Double Front Stroke (8 reps)

Huggers

Yoga Hamstring Stretch, with feet wide apart

Yoga Hamstring Stretch

Downward-Facing Dog

Standing Quad Stretch

Beginner's Yoga Routine

Begin every yoga practice by preparing a place that is free of clutter and helps you feel relaxed. You might light a candle or an incense stick, or put some flowers in a vase—anything to add to the serenity of the experience. Wear comfortable clothing, and place your yoga mat on the floor. Some people like to put on some soft, soothing music as well—you might try bamboo flute music, or sitar music like that of Ravi Shankar. Turn off cell phones, computers, spouses—anything that will distract you and spoil the tranquility of your yoga session. Don't force your body to stretch beyond its capacity. Take it easy, and stretch further as you become more flexible with regular practice.

There are 3 total rounds for this Beginner's routine. Start with your right side first, then repeat the sequence on your left to complete one round.

Mountain Pose

Side Stretch

Forward Bend

Yoga Hamstring Stretch

Flat Back (Partial Sun Salute)

Forward Bend

Plank

Chataranga

Upward-Facing Dog

Plank

Downward-Facing Dog

Runner's Pose

Warrior I

Warrior II

Bound Angle Pose (Baddha Konasana); final round only, hold for 5 breaths

Child's Pose; final round only, hold for 5 breaths

Corpse Pose (Savasana); final round only, hold for 10 breaths

Trainer's Tip: The last 3 moves are only performed at the end of the final round because they are intended for stretch and relaxation.

Sample Schedule for Beginners

I do want you to get in the habit of doing something active every day. Remember what I said about avoiding "exercise bipolar disorder"? If you want to feel good and make progress, daily activity is a must.

As a Beginner, this means only 20 minutes a day. Here is a sample training schedule for Beginners. If your schedule doesn't yet permit daily workouts, it's fine to double up; that is, do your cardio routine, followed by your resistance training or flexibility or a similar combination.

Monday:	Cardio training (20 minutes)
Tuesday:	Resistance training (20 minutes)
Wednesday:	Cardio training (20 minutes)
Thursday:	Resistance training (20 minutes)
Friday:	Yoga (20 minutes)
Saturday:	Resistance training (20 minutes)
Sunday:	Rest, do some yoga moves, or enjoy a fun sport that suits you, based on your Fun Factor results

Tony's Motivators: Winging It Won't Work

Schedule all your workouts in advance—at least a month ahead of time. This creates structure for your fitness plan and prevents you from prioritizing other things over fitness. You can use a simple paper calendar to schedule your workouts or, if you prefer, use your iPhone, Blackberry, or Outlook calendar—whatever works best for you. I met a guy, Steve, at one of my fitness camps who admitted he posted a paper calendar on his bathroom mirror, refrigerator, and even his front door! "I looked at the one on the fridge and I ignored it, but when I had one on my bathroom mirror and my front door, I was constantly reminded that my workouts had to be a priority in my life," he said.

I have a desk calendar that stares back at me all day long. After 25 years of training, I still write down the type of workout I've done and circle the day I did it. At the end of the month, I add them up. My goal (for the last 21 years) has been a minimum of 20 workouts a month—that's 240 a year with 125 days off.

I've always said that if you don't know what you're doing and when, you're toast. We're pretty good at scheduling when to wake up, when to go to bed, what time to eat, and when to watch our favorite shows, but for some reason we don't apply that same discipline to scheduling our workouts. The "I'll fit it in when I have spare time" philosophy just doesn't work. You can't create the healthy, fit life you want if you wing it. Soon, what was supposed to be Monday's workout becomes Tuesday's. Now Tuesday is on Wednesday and before you know it, it's Friday and you've barely worked out all week.

It's as simple as this: If you don't plan your workout, you probably won't do it. When you schedule your workouts in advance, your chances of success will skyrocket. My desk calendar has been a simple and effective tool for me for more than 20 years. Without it, I'm lost. With it, I'm organized, committed, and successful—and you will be, too.

That said, sometimes life intervenes and it becomes impossible to sustain or maintain your "perfect plan." Don't beat yourself up about it—you can't control everything. It's okay to miss a workout once in a while. It doesn't erase all of the hard work you've accomplished up until now or mean that you have to start over. Just pick up where you left off when you are able to. You will probably notice the difference between a missed workout or two and a missed week or two. If you miss one workout once in a while, you lose nothing. The extra day off can even do your body good. But if you miss a week or more, it will take you at least that long to get back to where you left off.

The more you plan and prepare, the better results you'll get.

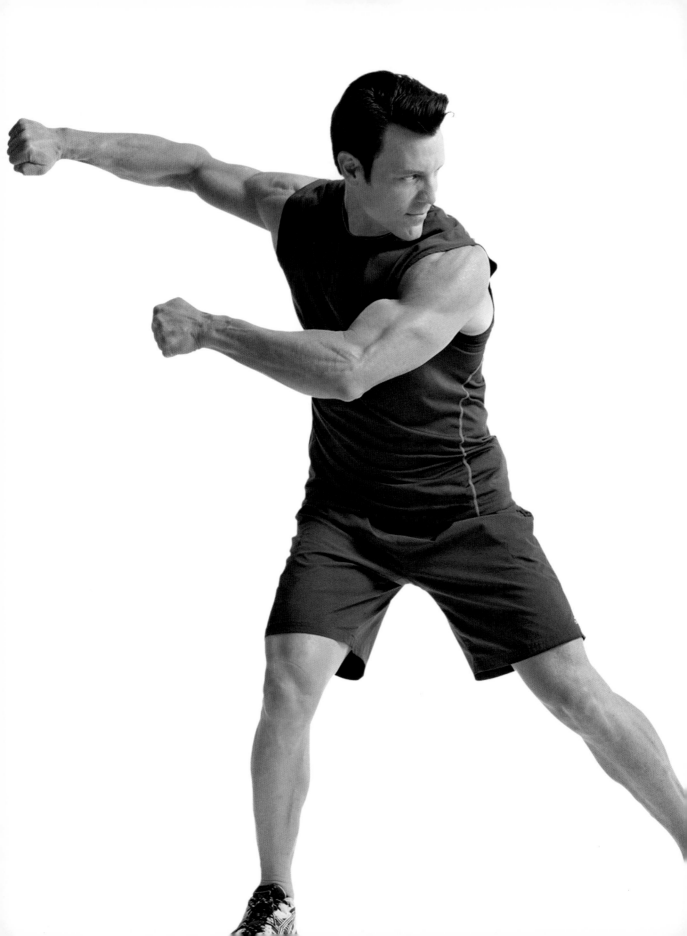

6

The Striver's Workout

For a Striver, consistency is going to be one of the single most critical components of getting in shape, burning fat, and staying fit and healthy. Why? Because up until now, you've possibly been sporadic in your workouts, and the results have come at a snail's pace, if at all. Or maybe you're semiregular at working out and need a new challenge to remotivate you. The Striver's workout will definitely take your toning, strength-building, and fat-burning to the next level.

Additional Equipment

In addition to resistance bands, an exercise bench, and a floor mat (see What You Need to Get Started on page 47), add the following equipment to your home gym:

Dumbbells. Buy a set of 5-, 8- and 10-pound dumbbells. You may need heavier weights later, but for now, these will work great.

Pullup bar. This piece of equipment is easy to install—you just slide it into any door frame. Try out different products before you buy one; look for sturdiness and high quality. Pullup bars, when used regularly and correctly, strengthen your chest, back, shoulders, and core, plus encourage great muscle development in the arms. Depending on where you place your hands on the pullup bar, you can isolate different muscle groups and feel the burn in different areas. I recommend the P90X Chin-Up Bar.

Your Leanest, Fittest Body Ever

With the Striver's workout, you'll work in circuits—continuous bouts of exercises that stoke your metabolism and build body-shaping muscle. Each pass through the circuit takes about 15 minutes, so with this workout, you'll increase the duration of your exercise sessions. Duration specifies how long to exercise at a single time. Since this workout is longer, you'll burn more calories and see toning results even sooner. By altering any aspect of your workout, such as duration, you will continue to progress.

And according to the independent test conducted by fitness coach Mark Briggs, you can burn 300 to 500 calories every time you do a Striver's workout. Just thinking about that caloric burn, plus the gains you're going to make in strength, muscular development, endurance, and general health, makes me want to hit the gym now!

The details: Striver's Phase 1 is approximately 35 minutes long; follow this workout for 3 weeks. Then switch to Striver's Phase 2—a workout that is approximately 40 minutes long and should be followed for another 3 weeks. After you've been consistent for 6 weeks, you will be ready to move on to the Warrior's workout.

If you have already completed the Beginner level, you'll be familiar with many of these exercises, though you'll also be adding a few different moves, plus some brand-new exercises that will increase the intensity and keep your workouts fun and interesting. When you keep challenging your muscles with new movements, they must constantly adapt, so results come quickly. As with all the workouts in this book, you'll be gaining cardiovascular endurance and developing strength and tone.

Some final notes: Be sure to do the prescribed warmups and cooldowns for each workout. Your General Warmup produces a gradual dilation of the blood vessels supplying the heart and skeletal muscles. This allows sufficient blood flow to the heart and skeletal muscles and reduces the risk of sudden increases in blood pressure. The Specific Warmups will include muscle stretches tailored to individual exercises. A gradual cooldown following the exercises will allow for a gradual reduction in heart rate and blood flow.

Remember: Only rest for about 30 seconds between sets, then get right back to work. That way, you'll keep your body on the move . . . and fat on the run.

Striver's Cardio Phase 1

General Warmup

March in place (30 steps)

Jog in place (40 steps)

Run in place (50 steps)

Jog in place (40 steps)

Specific Warmup

Side Stretch

Yoga Hamstring Stretch

Split-Leg Hamstring Stretch

Runner's Stretch

Downward-Facing Dog and pedal the feet (4 times per leg, and then static with both feet down for 4 breaths)

Standing Quad Stretch

The Workout (30 reps per move)

Circuit 1

Jumping Jacks

Line Leaps

Jab/Cross (15 combos on each side)

Leaping Lunges

Steam Engines

30-second rest, then repeat Circuit 1

30-second rest after repeating Circuit 1, then move to Circuit 2

Circuit 2

Pivot Punches

Lunge and Catch

Knee/Front Kicks (15 reps with each leg)

Briggs Ram

30-second rest and repeat circuit 2, then move to the Cooldown

Cooldown

March in place to bring down your heart rate (20 steps).

Side Stretch

Yoga Hamstring Stretch

Split-Leg Hamstring Stretch

Runner's Stretch

Downward-Facing Dog

Striver's Cardio Phase 2

General Warmup

Walk in place (30 steps)

Jog in place (40 steps)

Run in place (50 steps)

Specific Warmup

Side Stretch

Yoga Hamstring Stretch

Runner's Stretch

Downward-Facing Dog and pedal the feet (4 times per leg, and then static with both feet down for 4 breaths)

Standing Quad Stretch

The Workout (30 reps per move)

Circuit I

Pivot Twist (15 reps on each side)

Lateral Leaps

Jab/Cross/Hook/Uppercut (15 combos on each side)

High Knee Run

Steam Engines

Press Jacks

30-second rest, then repeat Circuit I

30-second rest after repeating Circuit I, then move to Circuit 2

Circuit 2

Pivot Punches

Lunge and Catch

Knee/Front Kicks (15 reps with each leg)

Briggs Ram

Lateral Lunge Reaches

30-second rest and repeat Circuit 2, then move to the Cooldown

Cooldown

March in place to bring down your heart rate (20 steps).

Side Stretch

Yoga Hamstring Stretch

Split-Leg Hamstring Stretch

Runner's Stretch

Downward-Facing Dog

Standing Quad Stretch

Striver's Resistance Phase I

General Warmup

Walk in place (30 steps)

Jog in place (40 steps)

Run in place (50 steps)

Specific Warmup

Head Rolls

Shoulder Rolls

Huggers

Yoga Hamstring Stretch, with feet wide apart

Yoga Hamstring Stretch

Downward-Facing Dog

Standing Quad Stretch

The Workout
Circuit 1

Standard Pushups, or from knees for Modified Pushups (max reps)

Lawnmowers (10–15 reps on each side)

Standing Swimmer's Presses (15–20 reps)

Standing Biceps Curls (10–15 reps)

Standing Double-Arm Triceps Presses (10–15 reps)

Shoulder-Width Squats (30–40 reps)

Bicycle (max reps)

30-second rest, then repeat Circuit 1

30-second rest after repeating Circuit 1, then move to Circuit 2

Circuit 2

Wide-Hand Pushups (max reps)

Bent-Over Rows (10–15 reps)

Upright Row Y-Presses, with dumbbells (10–15 reps)

21s

Wide-Feet Squats (30–40 reps)

In and Out Crunches (max reps)

30-second rest and repeat circuit 2, then move to the Cooldown

Cooldown

Shoulder Rolls

Chest Stretch

Side Stretch, with legs wide apart

Downward-Facing Dog

Standing Quad Stretch

Striver's Resistance Phase 2

General Warmup

Walk in place (30 steps)

Jog in place (40 steps)

Run in place (50 steps)

Jumping Jacks (20 reps)

Specific Warmup

Head Rolls

Shoulder Rolls

Huggers

Chest Stretch

Yoga Hamstring Stretch

Split-Leg Hamstring Stretch

Downward-Facing Dog

Flat Back (Partial Sun Salute)

The Workout

Circuit 1

Pullups (max reps)

Lawnmowers (15–20 reps on each side)

Standing Swimmer's Presses (15–20 reps)

Supinating Biceps Curls (10–15 reps)

Side Tri-Rises (10–15 reps on each side)

Plyometric Squats (20–30 reps)

Bicycle (30–50 reps)

30-second rest, then repeat Circuit 1

30-second rest after repeating Circuit 1, then move to Circuit 2

Circuit 2

Standard Pushups, or from knees for Modified Pushups (max reps)

Chinups (max reps)

Heavy Pants (10–15 reps)

Upright Rows (10–15 reps)

Crazy 8s (8 reps with each arm)

Palm Switch Grip Bent-Over Triceps Extensions (10–15 reps)

Wide-Feet Plyometric Squats (20–30 reps)

Scissor Crunches (20–30 reps)

30-second rest and repeat circuit 2, then move to the Cooldown

Cooldown

Huggers

Chest Stretch

Side Stretch

Yoga Hamstring Stretch

Split-Leg Hamstring Stretch

Striver's Yoga Routine

If you've diagnosed your fitness level as that of a Striver, or if you've been practicing the Beginner's Yoga Routine for about 3 weeks, the Striver's Yoga Routine is right for you. Its dynamic mix of poses—all performed while working to maintain balance—will leave you with supple muscles, a taller walk, and increased strength. I've introduced many new poses here. Getting into some of these poses isn't too difficult; the challenge is staying well-aligned and supported once you're there. Concentrate on using your muscles to do that.

Don't worry if it takes some time before you're able to make a fluid transition from one pose to the next. When I first started yoga, I struggled. I could barely touch my toes, and my limbs felt as though they weighed 500 pounds. But the benefits are cumulative, so the more you practice, the more flexibility and strength you achieve. Yoga also helps you build an awareness of your body, which will boost your self-image and confidence.

There are 3 total rounds for this Striver's routine. Start with your right side first, then repeat the sequence on your left to complete one round.

Mountain Pose

Side Stretch

Forward Bend

Yoga Hamstring Stretch

Flat Back (Partial Sun Salute)

Forward Bend

Plank

Chataranga

Upward-Facing Dog

Plank

Downward-Facing Dog

Runner's Pose

Warrior I

Warrior II

Reverse Warrior

Runner's Pose

Crescent Pose

Triangle Pose

Extended Right Angle Pose

Half Moon Pose

Bound Angle Pose (Baddha Konasana); final round only, hold for 5 breaths

Child's Pose; final round only, hold for 5 breaths

Corpse Pose (Savasana); final round only, hold for 10 breaths

Trainer's Tip: The last 3 moves are only performed at the end of the final round because they are intended for stretch and relaxation.

Sample Schedule for Strivers

Here is a sample training schedule for Strivers. If your schedule doesn't yet permit daily workouts, it's fine to double up; that is, do your cardio routine, followed by your resistance training or flexibility, or a similar combination.

Monday: Cardio training (35–40 minutes)

Tuesday: Resistance training (35–40 minutes)

Wednesday: Cardio training (35–40 minutes)

Thursday: Resistance training (35–40 minutes)

Friday: Yoga (35–40 minutes)

Saturday: Resistance training (35–40 minutes)

Sunday: Rest, do some yoga moves, or enjoy a fun sport that suits you, based on your Fun Factor results

Tony's Motivators: Find the Line!

The Line is that special place you need to get to if you want any program to work. It's the desire to do that extra pushup, to increase the depth and range of motion in your lunges and squats, to add more weight and resistance as you get stronger. It's discovering your pain/discomfort threshold so you can get the job done without jeopardizing good form or risking injury. If you undertrain or just plain give up because you "can't" do something the first few times, then you'll never know what it's like to be fit and healthy. Find the Line, do the best you can, and maintain good form.

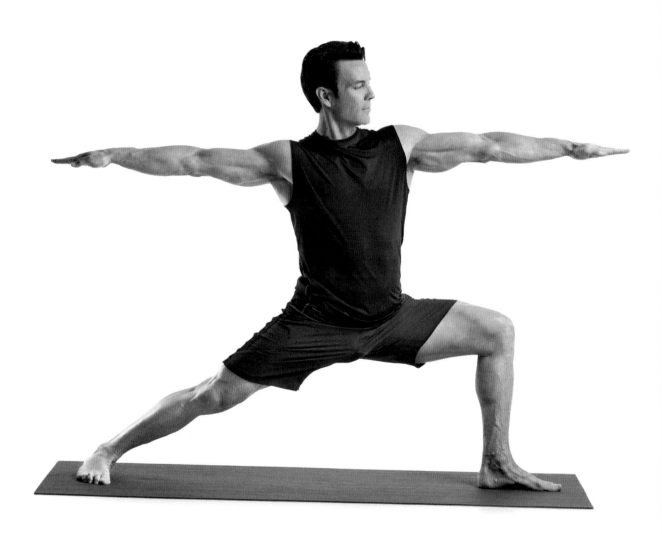

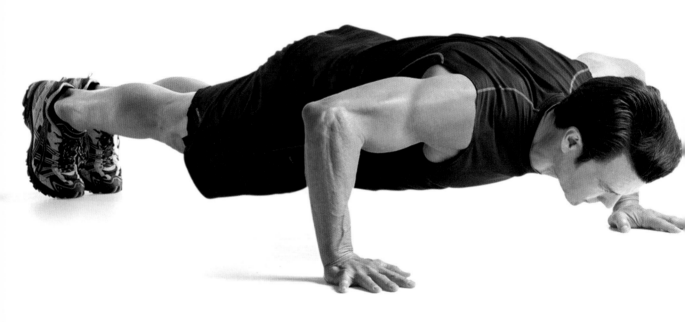

7

The Warrior's Workout

If you've made it to the Warrior level or are starting out there, congratulations! In the martial arts world, "warriors" have nearly superhuman skills. They can jump over an average person's head. They can break bricks. They have a ferocious training style, determination, and Zen-like focus. But most important, they can spend 8 hours a day, every day, working out. I'm not suggesting that at the Warrior level you do that, but if you can cultivate the heart of a warrior, it will redefine for you what it means to be strong, fit, and healthy.

I'm willing to bet that, until now, you've been wasting money on gym memberships and trainers who aren't giving you the results you've been looking for. Maybe you feel like you've been doing everything "right," but you're frustrated because you haven't seen the results you want. In the Warrior's workout, I'll show you how to burn fat and calories more efficiently; build long, lean, strong muscles; and become more flexible than you've ever been. All in less than 55 minutes a day! That's right: I want you to get it done in under an hour.

To continually progress, remember that muscles need overload and variety. You can overload a muscle with increased resistance, less rest, more sets, and/or more or different exercises.

The Warrior workouts won't just help you drop 10 pounds. These workouts are going to make you look forward to exercising. That's because each day brings a different workout, and this change-it-up strategy puts your body on the fast track to becoming firm and fit.

Additional Equipment

In addition to resistance bands, an exercise bench, and a floor mat (see What You Need to Get Started on page 47), include the following equipment in your home gym. If you've completed the Striver level, you already have most of these.

Pullup bar: An exercise bar that you can install by placing and securing it in a door frame.

BOSU ball: An exercise device that looks like a stability ball that has been cut in half. It has an inflated dome on one side and is flat on the other.

Medicine ball: An exercise ball that is sold in a variety of weights and sizes (typically ranging from 2 to 20 pounds).

Your pattern for advancement will be the same as with the Beginner and Striver levels: two phases of cardio and resistance workouts. There's a Warrior's Yoga Routine, too. Each workout is faster paced, more intense, longer in duration, and filled with new moves.

The Warrior's Bonus Round

One of the greatest things about being a Beginner is the rapid pace at which you make gains. During your first few weeks of training, strength and muscular gains come quickly and relatively easily. If only those gains could continue indefinitely! When you reach Warrior status, you really have to change things up to take your fitness level up a notch and keep progressing.

You have a number of options to keep you from hitting a plateau: You can adjust the frequency of your workouts (work out more often), modify the volume of your work (work out harder), or change the exercise program itself (work out differently). You can also make significant changes to your workout by learning new exercises and mixing up the order in which you do them. The Warrior's Bonus Round will show you how to do this.

And if you want to increase the duration of your resistance workout, simply add in the Bonus Round. By varying your routine in any number of ways, you can deliver growth-inducing stimulus.

An Amazing Calorie Burn

Warriors: Here's where you can burn a crazy number of calories. Fitness coach Mark Briggs found that during the 55-minute Warrior's workout, a person can burn up to 1,000 calories. A *thousand calories* in 55 minutes? The only exercise I know of that can do that is jumping rope—and who wants to do that for almost an hour, even though it's certainly a great way to get in shape.

Of course, to achieve the 1,000-calorie burn, you'd have to keep your pace of intensity at an all-time high: short rest periods, heavier resistance, all-out cardio on the cardio workouts, and so forth. But if you are able to burn 1,000 calories per workout and you work out every day, you can potentially knock off close to a pound of fat every 3 days.

But fat loss is just one of the benefits you'll see after training at Warrior level. You'll also improve your endurance, increase your energy, boost your heart health, and achieve the level of fitness and health you've been dreaming about for years.

Warrior's Cardio Phase I

General Warmup

March in place (40 steps)

Jog in place (50 steps)

Run in place (60 steps)

Jumping Jacks (30 reps)

Specific Warmup

Side Stretch

Yoga Hamstring Stretch to the center

Runner's Stretch

Downward-Facing Dog

Flat Back (Partial Sun Salute) (3 times)

Standing Quad Stretch

The Workout

Circuit 1

Wide-Feet Squats (30 reps)

Runner's Lunge/Knee Pulls (15 reps on each side)

Back Lunge/Front Kicks (20 reps with each leg)

Fast Feet Football Drill (20 reps)

Jab/Cross/Hook/Uppercut (20 reps on each side—each set of 4 punches counts as 1 rep)

Run Kicks (30 reps)

30-second rest, then repeat Circuit 1

30-second rest after repeating Circuit 1, then move to Circuit 2

Circuit 2

Wacky Jacks (50 reps)

Fighter Squats (30 reps, switch lead foot every rep)

Lunge Jumps (30 reps)

Double Back Hammer/Front Kicks (30 reps, alternating right and left)

Deep Lateral Leaps (30 reps)

30-second rest and repeat Circuit 2, then move to the Cooldown

Cooldown

Jog in place to bring down your heart rate (30 steps).

Side Stretch

Yoga Hamstring Stretch

Split-Leg Hamstring Stretch

Runner's Stretch

Downward-Facing Dog

Standing Quad Stretch

Warrior's Cardio Phase 2

General Warmup

Jog in place (40 steps)

Run in place (50 steps)

Sprint in place (60 steps)

Specific Warmup

Side Stretch

Yoga Hamstring Stretch to the center

Runner's Stretch

Downward-Facing Dog

Flat Back (Partial Sun Salute) (3 times)

Standing Quad Stretch

The Workout

Circuit 1

Sprint Squats (25 reps)

Lunge Kicks (30 reps)

Steam Engine Kicks (40 reps)

Jack-in-the-Box Jump Squats (20 reps)

Jab/Cross/Hook/Uppercut/Knee/Front Kick (15 reps on each side—each set of
4 punches and knee/kick combo counts as 1 rep)

Standing Speed Climbers (50 reps)

30-second rest, then repeat Circuit 1

30-second rest after repeating Circuit 1, then move to Circuit 2

Circuit 2

Jump Knee Tucks/Low Squat Hops (12 reps)

Lateral Leap Kicks (25 reps)

Double Lunge/Double Squat Switches (12 reps)

High Knee Run (30 reps)

Double Jab/Low Punch/Kick (12 combos on each side)

Burpee Sprints (15 reps)

30-second rest and repeat Circuit 2, then move to the Cooldown

Cooldown

Jog in place to bring down your heart rate (30 steps).

Side Stretch

Yoga Hamstring Stretch

Split-Leg Hamstring Stretch

Runner's Stretch

Downward-Facing Dog

Standing Quad Stretch

Warrior's Resistance Phase I

General Warmup

March in place (25 steps)

Jog in place (35 steps)

Run in place (45 steps)

Jumping Jacks (40 reps)

Specific Warmup

Head Rolls

Shoulder Rolls

Arm Circles

Huggers

Chest Stretch

Yoga Hamstring Stretch

Split-Leg Hamstring Stretch

Runner's Stretch

Downward-Facing Dog

The Workout

Circuit I

Wide-Hand Pullups (max reps)

Lawnmowers (10–12 reps on each side)

In and Out Biceps Curls (10–12 reps)

One Arm (Behind the Head) Triceps Extensions (8–10 reps)

Plyometric Squats (30–40 reps)

Tick Tock Lifts (20 reps)

Wide-Hand and Leg Pushups (max reps)

Knee-Up Chinups (max reps)

Straight-Arm Posterior Delt Flies (10–12 reps)

Upright Rows (8–10 reps)

21s

Bent-Over Switch-Grip Triceps Extensions (10–15 reps)

Wide-Feet Squats (30–40 reps)

Bicycle, in fast motion (75–100 reps)

30-second rest, then repeat Circuit I

30-second rest after repeating Circuit I, then move to the Bonus Round!

Bonus Round

Pushup Jacks (max reps)

Switch-Grip Pullups, 2 reps overgrip / 2 reps undergrip (max reps)

Pike Presses with Leg Raise (max reps)

Crazy 8s (32 total reps)

Chuck-Ups—3 hand positions with isometric hold at top and bottom
    (4 reps each—12 total)

Chair Frog Squats (30–40 reps)

Bicycle (20–30 reps)

Cooldown

Head Rolls

Shoulder Rolls

Side Stretch

Runner's Stretch

Downward-Facing Dog

Warrior's Resistance Phase 2

General Warmup

March in place (25 steps)

Jog in place (35 steps)

Run in place (45 steps)

Jumping Jacks (40 reps)

Specific Warmup

Head Rolls

Shoulder Rolls

Arm Circles

Huggers

Chest Stretch

Yoga Hamstring Stretch

Split-Leg Hamstring Stretch

Runner's Stretch

Downward-Facing Dog

The Workout

For one-legged moves, change foot with each rep

Circuit I

Chuck-Ups (20 reps)

Wide-to-Narrow Pullups (max reps)

One-Foot Rear Delt Flies with Band (8 reps on each foot)

Standing Shoulder Presses, balancing on one foot (8 reps on each foot)

Alternating Biceps Curls

Split-Leg Side Tri-Rises (max reps on each side)

Speed Squats (50–60 reps, switch weight-bearing leg every 5th rep)

Banana Crunches (20 reps)

Circuit 2

Rami Plyo Pushups (max reps)

Chinups (max reps)

One-Foot Curl and Press (8–12 reps on each foot)

Shoulder Flies on One Foot (4–6 reps on each foot)

Bent-Over 21s

Bent-Over Switch-Grip Triceps Extensions—balancing on one foot (10–12 reps palms up on right foot, then 10–12 palms down on left)

Screamer Lunges (30 reps, alternating legs)

Side-Arm-Balance Crunches (20–30 reps on each side)

Circuit 3

Pushup Jacks (max reps)

Levers (max reps)

Two-Ball Pike Presses (max reps)

Alternating Biceps Curls (8–12 reps)

Side Tri-Rises (max reps)

Wall Squats (3 minutes or more)

In-Out-Up-Down-Open-Close (15 reps)

Cooldown

Head Rolls

Shoulder Rolls

Side Stretch

Runner's Stretch

Downward-Facing Dog

Warrior's Yoga Routine

If you have done yoga before, this routine will deepen your yoga practice. I've chosen additional poses that will stretch and challenge your balance.

If you have not done much or any yoga before, try the Beginner's or Striver's yoga routines first to get a feel for this wonderful activity. Because your body is strong, I'm willing to bet that you can quickly start incorporating some of these more advanced moves into your practice.

Once you get the hang of it, I encourage you to stick to this routine. The physical and mental changes you experience will surprise and inspire you. Yoga is a journey of the heart and soul and an opening of the body's energy channels to receive all of life's gifts.

There are 3 total rounds for this Warrior's routine. Start with your right side first, then repeat the sequence on your left to complete one round.

Mountain Pose

Side Stretch

Forward Bend

Yoga Hamstring Stretch

Flat Back (Partial Sun Salute)

Forward Bend

Plank

Chataranga with Leg Raise

Upward-Facing Dog

Plank

Downward-Facing Dog

Runner's Pose

Warrior I

Warrior II

Reverse Warrior

Runner's Pose

Crescent Pose

Triangle Pose

Extended Right Angle Pose

Half Moon Pose

Mountain Pose

Standing Leg Extension

Crane Pose

Advanced Forward Bend Hamstring Stretch

Pigeon

Advanced Runner's Pose (see Advanced Runner's Stretch on page 187)

Bound Angle Pose (Baddha Konasana); final round only, hold for 5 breaths

Child's Pose; final round only, hold for 5 breaths

Corpse Pose (Savasana); final round only, hold for 10 breaths

Trainer's Tip: The last 3 moves are only performed at the end of the final round because they are intended for stretch and relaxation.

Sample Schedule for Warriors

Here is a sample training schedule for Warriors. If your schedule doesn't permit daily workouts, it's fine to double up; that is, do your cardio routine, followed by your resistance training or flexibility, or a similar combination.

Monday:	Cardio training (55 minutes)
Tuesday:	Resistance training (55 minutes)
Wednesday:	Cardio training (55 minutes)
Thursday:	Resistance training (55 minutes)
Friday:	Yoga (55 minutes)
Saturday:	Resistance training (55 minutes)
Sunday:	Rest, do some yoga moves, or enjoy a fun sport that suits you, based on your Fun Factor results

Tony's Motivators: Do Your Best and Forget the Rest

I fall in love with any maxim, motto, proverb, aphorism, or truism that keeps me focused and inspired, and one of my favorites is "Do your best and forget the rest." When I ask you to do your best and forget the rest, I'm asking you to show up and be okay with how you're doing right now, rather than compare yourself to the previous time. The place and head space you're in right now are all you have. Why would you want to ruin it by comparing it to something else?

If a particular workout seems too daunting, or if you don't feel like doing it, it's also okay to skip parts of a workout or substitute moves. Run in place if you don't feel like doing plyometrics, for example. I'm here to tell you that it's perfectly okay to cheat, take breaks, and skip some moves if that's what you need to do to get through a workout. I do this all the time.

As much as I want you to "Find the Line" and push your limits, some days doing your best can also mean pushing yourself a little. When I'm trying to bust through a plateau, I'll add just one more rep to each set—that's all. It's paying off because my strength and power have improved immensely. I've been an 8- or 10-rep guy forever, so my body and mind have adapted. I've been in unwanted maintenance mode. No more! Instead of upping the weight to create more resistance (sometimes causing joint pain and injury), I'm just adding the extra rep whenever I can. Turning 8 reps to 9 and 10 to 11 has been surprisingly hard, but the results are undeniable. If you're in a rut, then just add a rep whenever and wherever you can. It's that simple. It will help you avoid boredom, injury, and plateaus, plus speed up your results.

And if you take exercise classes, don't get caught up in the collective energy of the room. Do your best and forget the rest! If at any point in the workout you find that there is something that you can't physically do, modify the movement or run or jog in place.

Any workout is always better than no workout at all. When you shift your mind to doing *something* (even when you don't want to), you'll be less likely to completely fall off the fitness wagon. Don't let your ego fight what's happening to you right now. Gracefully accept the conditions that present themselves as opposed to fighting the reality of your situation. Go with your flow, based on who you are right now, and stop fighting the truth of now because you so desperately want to keep up with your past. If you can do this and accept this, then you'll know how to stay fit and healthy for the rest of your life. I'm told other good maxims to live by include "Look both ways before you cross the street" and "Don't take candy from a stranger." I need to do further research on these, so in the meantime, I'm sticking with "Do your best and forget the rest."

PART 3 The Moves

You've arrived at the part of the book where I show you how to do my exclusive workouts, using detailed instructions and step-by-step photographs. Now that you've assessed your level of fitness and identified the routine that's right for you, it's time to learn how to do the exercises described in your new regimen. Whether you're a Beginner, Striver, or Warrior, read through the exercises first, then try doing each one so you can begin to master it. If there's a move or exercise that's out of your comfort zone, it's okay to skip it (for now) or modify it to your fitness level. In some cases, I'll recommend modifications for you. It's important to listen to your body and understand that trying to keep up for the sake of keeping up is counterproductive. Remember: Do your best and forget the rest.

If you practice the exercises as described and follow your plan closely, you'll notice dramatic improvements in your strength, endurance, and stamina within a few weeks. If you have a bad day here and there, don't beat yourself up: Who cares if you could do 40 pushups last week and today you can do only 30? It happens. It just is. Are you doing your best? If you are and your numbers aren't as great as last time, you're still exactly where you need to be.

My program is designed and calibrated to keep you "off balance" just enough so that you don't settle into a plateau. Most other programs stop working after a while because the body falls into a rut. Not this program. My workouts have a built-in rut-breaking system. Each routine allows room for improvement. Over time, you get better and better, regardless of what happens during an individual workout. Just stay intense, stay consistent, and have fun!

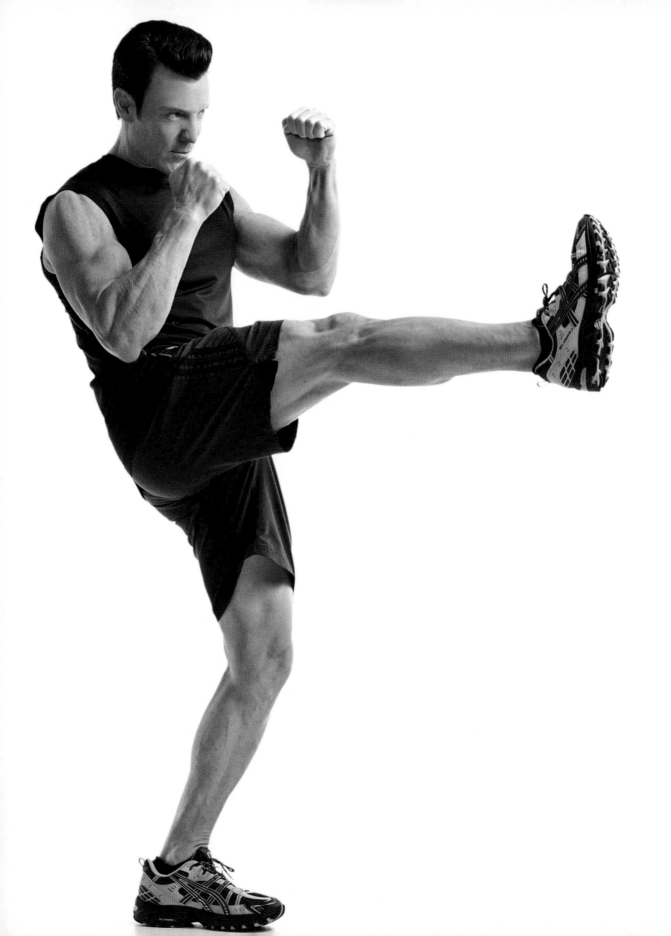

8

Cardio Fat Burners

This chapter is for cardio haters like me. Yes, I dread cardio, but I know I have to do it. What works for me—and what will work for you—is the following: First, variety. I have to mix it up. If I have access to machines, I'll do 5 to 10 minutes on each, and those might include moving laterally on a Slide Board, vertically on a VersaClimber or stair stepper, and linearly on a stationary bike or treadmill. That way, I don't get bored. Plus, I'm less likely to get injured because I'm not doing the same monotonous move over and over again. I don't like to go on long runs much because I have the average attention span of a gnat on eight cups of coffee. I need to constantly change things up.

I've also been known to create my very own cardio obstacle course at home—and you can, too. Try jogging in place for 5 to 10 minutes, followed by some high-knee raises for another stretch, then walk up and down a flight of stairs. Follow that by cranking up some lively music with a great beat and dancing. Voilà—there you have a cardio routine you can do in your house for 20 minutes or more and reap its aerobic benefits. Even at 52, I still dance around the house like a teenager once in a while. (Robot, anyone?)

The second way to make cardio more bearable is brevity. You've probably been told that you have to do cardio three times a week for the best results. That's fine, and you can do that. But here's the truth: Doing cardio at least twice a week is effective, and that's what I do. The routines in this book are set up to include twice-a-week cardio, but if you'd like to do more, go for it.

The third and final way to get on better terms with cardio is the most powerful (and the main) reason I do it: its effect on your brain and your mood. Cardio, for sure, is about fat burning, kicking your metabolism into high gear, and changing the shape of your butt and your legs. But first and foremost for me, cardio positively affects the quality of my life. It makes sense when you think about it. Working out helps keep your muscles and bones in shape. So doesn't it seem to follow that working out should keep your brain fit, too?

That's exactly what researchers at the University of Texas Southwestern Medical Center at Dallas proved when they put 5,451 men and 1,277 women (ages 20 to 88) on a weekly program of walking, jogging, and running, plus a treadmill test. For every 11 to 19 miles they logged each week, their mental health improved. They had fewer symptoms of depression, better moods, and much improved emotional health.[1]

One of the main reasons for all these mood-boosting benefits is that your brain releases chemicals (endorphins) while you exercise that relax the body and release tension. And if endorphins aren't enough, the positive effects of cardio on your body definitely will lift your spirits.

Cardio also helps with stress management. Stress is harmful to your mind and body and can lead to illnesses like high blood pressure, heart disease, ulcers, and migraines, and mental health problems like chronic anxiety and difficulty managing anger. Exercise burns off excess energy and adrenaline generated by stress and produces feel-good hormones called endorphins that help lift your mood.

Cardio also helps lift depression. While everyone gets the blues at one time or another, some people experience intense bouts of depression for prolonged periods of time. Left unresolved, depression can sap your energy, suppress your libido, hinder your ability to concentrate, bring on sleep disorders, suppress your immune system, and hamper your enjoyment of life.

Consider Emily, a New York City resident who has used P90X.

Emily was 49 when she lost her mother, aunt, and uncle in the same year.

"I spent the following summer sitting on the couch, eating all day," she says. "I felt overwhelmed, stressed, sad, and full of grief. I had given up."

A chiropractor convinced Emily to give one of my at-home programs a try. Though intimidated at first, she stepped up to the plate. "It was hard in the beginning," she admits. "But I refused to give up. And then the magic happened. The stronger I got, the better I felt." Today she says, "My body, mind, and spirit are in the best places they've ever been. I couldn't be healthier—or happier."

You can experience the same mood-altering effects that Emily did. The bottom line is that cardio fortifies you for life.

Now, if cardio is a 7-day-a-week passion for you, you've also come to the right place. I'm going to give you a whole new approach to aerobic exercise that most people have never heard of. You'll learn brand-new moves that don't involve the elliptical machine, stationary bike, or treadmill. Not that there is anything wrong with these expensive, space-consuming cardio machines, if you like repetitive movements and boredom. My style of cardio is designed around three types of aerobic exercise: Kenpo, plyometrics, and super cardio moves.

Kenpo

When I was 20 years old, I decided to take a martial arts class in Santa Monica. It just happened to be Kenpo karate, a streetwise martial art. If you're an Elvis Presley fan, you would know this form of karate, because Elvis interjected Kenpo movements into his concert performances during the latter part of his career. All the adult classes available at the time were geared toward people who already had some martial arts experience, so I—a complete newbie—enrolled in a kids' class. I stayed in the class for 6 months and couldn't believe how many great moves I was learning—and how well I fit in with 7-year-olds. Even better, I was amazed by how I started feeling.

Kenpo and other martial arts–based workouts change the focus from how you look to what your body can do. Put another way, the martial arts give you something to focus on instead of being body conscious. In the classes I took, I didn't ask myself, "How do I look?" I asked, "What am I made of?" The energy I released and the stamina I built during those hard-core workouts inspired me to take control of my life. Control is a large part of the appeal of Kenpo for me. There's so much in life we can't control, but in the workout arena, we control and use specific forms of conditioning to restructure our bodies and minds. Much has been written about the mind's influence on the body. Yet it works the other way, too: The body has a tremendous influence on the mind.

The word *Kenpo* means "Law of the Fist" (an ancient precursor to "Talk to the Hand"), and that's exactly what you'll be throwing during these fun, skill-based, cardio-intense moves. With the possible exception of *earlobe*, you name a body part, you'll be using it. Kenpo, by the way, includes more than just the standard kickboxing stuff you've probably tried in the past. Although kickboxing is a great workout, you can get bored with it. Throwing punches into empty air loses its appeal after a while—at least, it did for me.

Kenpo is a full-body, *skill-building* workout using the philosophy of the martial arts. You'll work your hips, legs, upper body, core—all of it, in one heck of a total-body cardio workout. You'll also use a very dynamic range of motion that will improve your mobility and flexibility. And much like yoga, Kenpo involves a combination of moves that are very functionally based, so while you're improving your aerobic power and burning fat, you're also developing your coordination, hand-eye movement, balance, and stamina. Kenpo has always challenged me personally, so while I was developing the cardio segments of my at-home workouts, I decided to incorporate Kenpo into all my aerobic routines. I hope you enjoy it as much as I do.

My Kenpo Moves

Jab/Cross

Start: Take a fighter's stance, with your knees slightly bent and your head facing forward. Your feet should be about shoulder-width apart, with your right foot behind your left and your right heel off the ground. Your elbows should be close to your sides and your hands held in the fighter's stance.

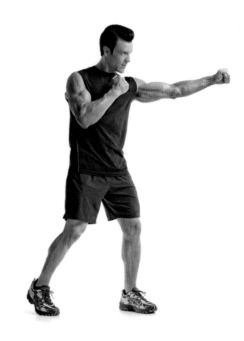

Action: Punch with your forward arm straight out in front of you.

Then, as you begin to retract your hand to the start position, punch forward (slightly across the center-line of your body) with your other hand. As you punch, rotate your rear hip in the direction of the punch. (This is what generates the power of the punch.)

Repeat the entire sequence for the designated number of repetitions, then switch the lead foot and repeat on the opposite side.

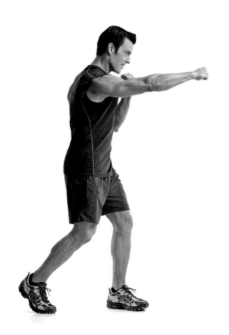

Jab/Cross/Hook/ Uppercut Sequence

Start: Take a fighter's stance, with your knees slightly bent and your head facing forward. Your feet should be about shoulder-width apart, with your right foot behind your left and your right heel off the ground. Your elbows should be close to your sides and your hands held in the fighter's stance.

Action: Punch with your forward arm straight out in front of you, then as you begin to retract your hand to the start position, punch forward (slightly across the centerline of your body) with your other hand. As you punch, rotate your rear hip in the direction of the punch.

Next, you will throw the hook punch using your lead hand. Pull your lead hand back slightly, then swing your fist in a horizontal looping motion (envision clearing items off the top of a table). As you punch, rotate the toes of your front foot slightly in the direction of the punch, enabling you to slightly turn your hip at the same time.

Return your hand to the start position and quickly lower your rear hand toward your waist, bending your back knee slightly at the same time. Spring upright as you deliver the uppercut, swinging your rear hand up as if to strike an opponent under the chin.

Repeat the entire sequence for the designated number of repetitions, then switch legs and repeat on the opposite side.

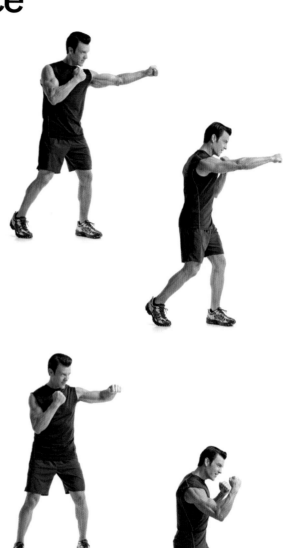

Jab/Cross/Hook/Uppercut/Knee/Front Kick

Start: Take a fighter's stance, with your knees slightly bent and your head facing forward. Your feet should be about shoulder-width apart, with your right foot behind your left and your right heel off the ground. Your elbows should be close to your sides and your hands held in the fighter's stance.

Action: Punch with your forward arm straight out in front of you, then as you begin to retract your hand to the start position, punch forward (slightly across the centerline of your body) with your other hand. As you punch, rotate your rear hip in the direction of the punch.

Next, you will throw the hook punch using your lead hand. Pull your lead hand back slightly, then swing your fist in a horizontal looping motion (envision clearing items off the top of a table). As you punch, rotate the toes of your front foot slightly in the direction of the punch, enabling you to slightly turn your hip at the same time.

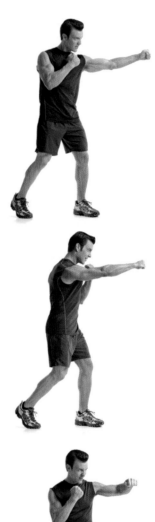

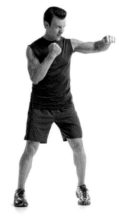

Return your hand to the start position. Quickly lower your rear hand toward your waist, and swing it in an upward motion (as if striking an opponent under the chin). As your hand moves toward your waist, bend your back knee slightly, and then spring back upright as you deliver the uppercut.

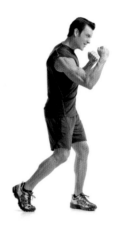

Immediately upon completion of the uppercut, throw a knee strike with your back leg.

Reset your leg, and then throw a front kick.

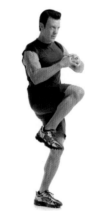

Repeat the entire sequence for the designated number of repetitions, then switch legs and repeat on the opposite side.

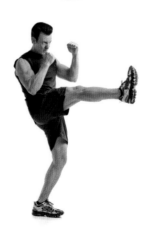

Pivot Punches

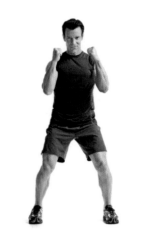

Start: Stand facing forward with your feet more than shoulder-width apart and your knees slightly bent. Your heels and toes should be in alignment. Your elbows should be close to the sides of your body, and your hands should be held close to your chin, with fists clenched.

Action: Begin by twisting your body to the left, making sure to rotate on your toes so that both feet also face to the left. As you twist, throw a strong punch to the left with your right hand.

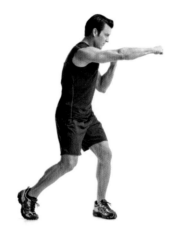

Quickly change directions and repeat on the opposite side, making sure this time to punch with your left hand. This should be a fast, fluid motion. Continue alternating arms for the designated number of repetitions.

Speed Pivot Punch Variation: Perform the Pivot Punches as described above, but with increased speed and punching intensity.

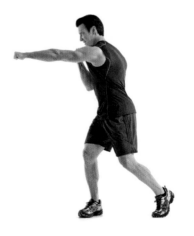

Front Kicks

Start: Stand in a fighter's stance, with your knees slightly bent and your head facing forward. Your feet should be about 12 inches apart, your back heel off the ground, and your weight balanced on the balls of both feet.

Action: While maintaining your fighter's stance, kick forward with your back leg, flexing your toes back. Envision striking an opponent with the ball of the foot on your kicking leg. Return to the start position, and repeat for the designated number of repetitions. Switch legs and repeat on the opposite side.

Note: Make sure to keep some flexion in the kicking leg so that you don't lock your knee, risking injury through hyperextension.

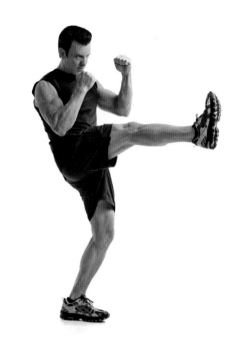

Knee/Front Kicks

Start: Stand with your knees slightly bent and your head facing forward. Your feet should be about 12 inches apart. Lift your right knee up toward your chest.

Action: Kick forward with your right leg, flexing your toes back, and envision striking an opponent with the ball of the foot on your kicking leg.

Repeat for the designated number of repetitions, then switch legs and repeat on the opposite side.

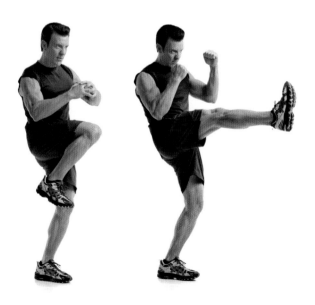

Back Lunge/Front Kicks

Start: Stand with your feet about shoulder-width apart and your knees relaxed. Bend your elbows to bring your forearms up in front of your chest for balance.

Action: Step back into a lunge, making sure to keep your front knee over your ankle and your back leg straight.

Quickly push off your back leg to return to a standing position, and follow through into a front kick (using the same leg you stepped back into the lunge with).

Repeat for the designated number of repetitions, then switch legs and repeat on the opposite side.

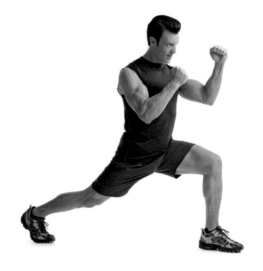

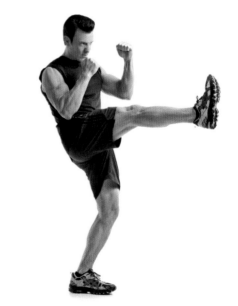

Run Kicks

Start: Begin running in place with your hands up in the fighter's stance.

Action: Lean back slightly and continue running, lifting your knees higher as you run. Kick forward with your right leg.

Kick forward with your left leg.

Raise your arms slightly and run in place.

Hop up once.

Repeat the sequence for the designated number of repetitions, alternating legs with every kick.

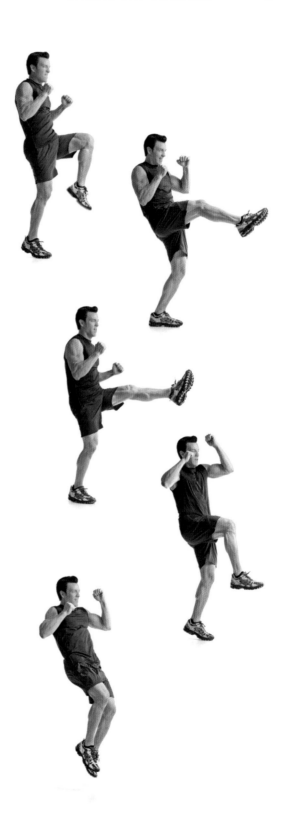

Fighter Squats

Start:
Take the fighter's stance, with your knees slightly bent, one foot in front of the other, and your head facing forward. Your feet should be about hip-width apart, your weight on the balls of both feet. Your elbows should be close to your sides and your hands held in the fighter's stance.

Action:
Squat down in the fighter's stance; then return to the start position. Switch lead feet and repeat on the opposite side. Continue alternating for the designated number of repetitions.

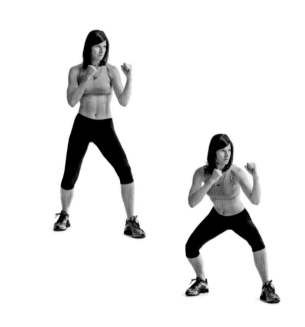

Lunge Kicks

Start:
With your left leg, step forward into a lunge position. Your right leg should be extended behind you.

Action:
Rock back on your right leg and kick up your left leg.

After kicking, switch legs and repeat on the other side to complete 1 repetition. Continue alternating legs for the designated number of repetitions.

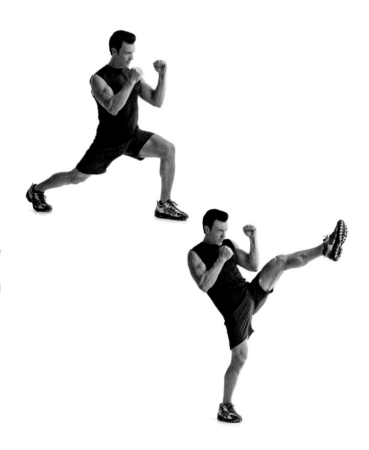

Double Jab/Low Punch/Kick

Start: Take the fighter's stance, with your knees slightly bent, one foot in front of the other, and your head facing forward. Your feet should be about 12 inches apart, your weight on the balls of both feet.

Action: Extend your left arm straight out in front of you and keep your right arm bent and close to your side.

Bring your left arm in close to your left side while simultaneously punching downward with your right fist.

Rock your body up and back, bring both arms to the fighter's position in front of your face, and kick vigorously forward with your right leg.

Switch legs and repeat on the opposite side. Continue alternating for the designated number of repetitions.

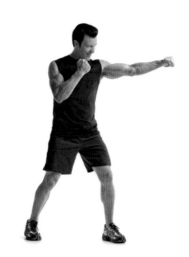

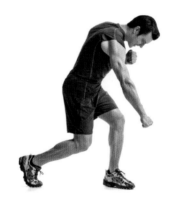

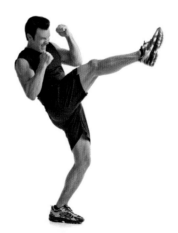

Double Back Hammer/Front Kicks

Start: Take the fighter's stance, as shown.

Action: With your left leg forward and right leg back, simultaneously back-fist punch your left hand in front of you and your right hand behind you.

Quickly return to the start position and throw a front snap kick with your right foot.

Return to the start position and repeat the entire sequence for the designated number of repetitions, then switch legs and repeat on the opposite side.

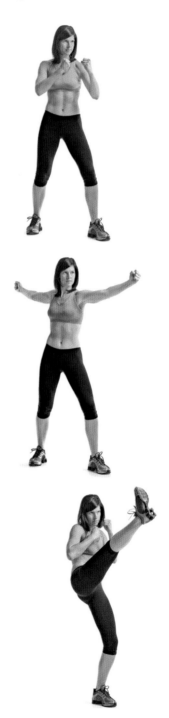

My Plyometric Moves

Note: Whenever doing any type of plyometric leg exercise that requires you to bend down, always keep your core engaged and your knees bent as low as possible while keeping your head and chest up to prevent back injury.

Line Leaps

Start: Begin with your feet about shoulder-width apart and your arms bent at your sides.

Action: Picture a line on the floor directly in front of you. Keeping your feet shoulder-width apart, hop or skip forward over the imaginary line.

Then hop or skip backward over it to complete 1 rep.

Repeat for the designated number of repetitions.

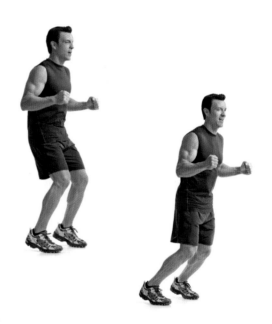

Lateral Leaps

Start: Stand with your feet about shoulder-width apart and your arms at your sides.

Action: Jump to the right, landing on your right foot with your left leg raised slightly.

Jump to your left, landing on your left foot with your right leg raised slightly, to complete 1 rep.

Repeat for the designated number of repetitions.

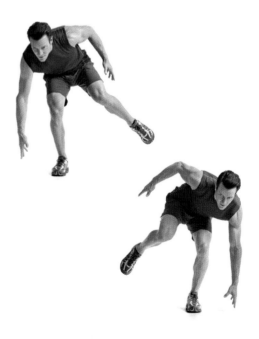

Lateral Leap Kicks

Start: Stand with your feet about 12 inches apart. Hold your arms in a fighter's stance. Lift your right knee.

Action: Leap to the right and land on your right foot, then do a front snap kick with your left leg.

Repeat in the opposite direction to complete 1 rep, then continue the entire sequence for the designated number of repetitions.

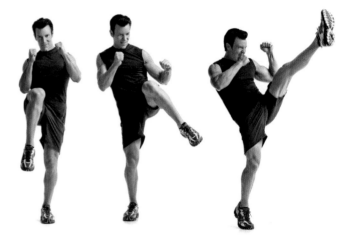

Deep Lateral Leaps

Start: Stand in a deep squat with your feet slightly separated and your fingertips touching the floor just outside of your feet.

Action: Explosively jump up laterally to your right, reaching overhead as you jump.

Land with your feet together and repeat in the opposite direction to complete 1 rep, then continue the entire sequence for the designated number of repetitions.

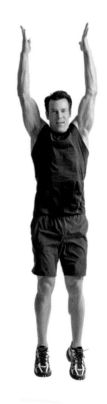

Chair Frog Squats

Start: Stand with your feet and knees together in a squat, arms overhead, and weight in your heels (imagine that you're sitting in a chair).

Action: While remaining low, jump your feet out and bring your fingertips to the floor in front of you (keep your head and chest up while maintaining a low squat position).

Jump back to the start position and repeat for the designated number of repetitions.

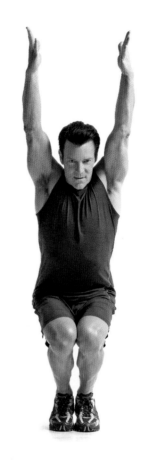

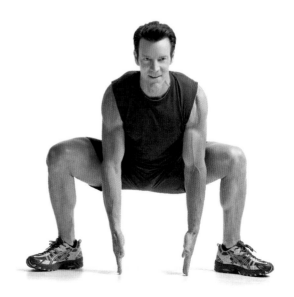

Pushup Jacks

Start: Assume the standard pushup position: feet behind you but positioned slightly more than shoulder-width apart. Place your hands about 2 to 3 feet apart.

Action: Lower your body to the floor and simultaneously jump your legs apart.

As you push back up to the start position, simultaneously jump your feet together.

Repeat for the designated number of repetitions.

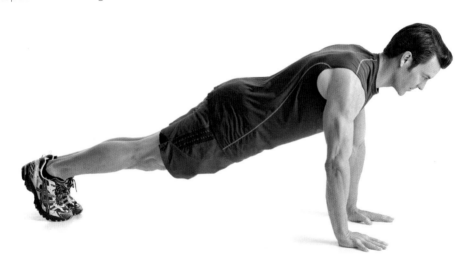

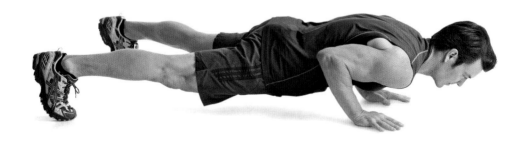

Double Lunge/
Double Squat Switches

Start: Position yourself with your right leg forward, left leg back, and hands up by your chest.

Action: Jump and switch your feet in the lunge position (left leg forward), then jump into a squat position (performing 2 low jumping squats).

Jump back into a lunge with your right leg forward and repeat the entire sequence for the designated number of repetitions.

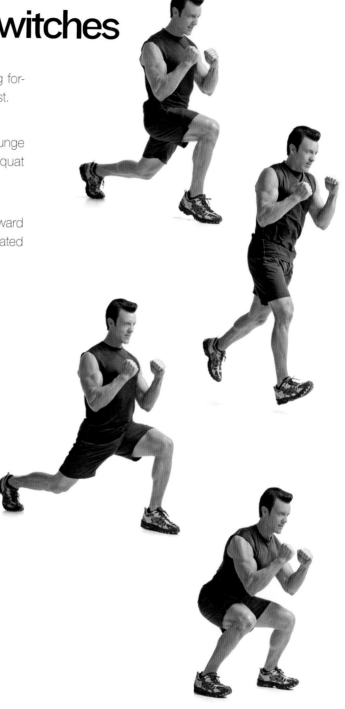

Lunge Jumps

Start: Bend both knees and crouch to the ground, with your right knee slightly in front of your left one.

Action: Jump upward, bringing your hands up above your head. Land with your left knee slightly in front of your right one. Repeat to return to the start position. Repeat the sequence for the designated number of repetitions.

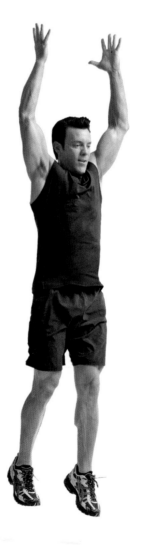

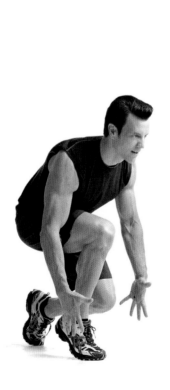

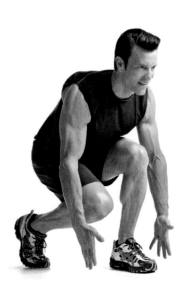

Leaping Lunges

Start: Place your left foot in front of you and your right foot behind you. Keeping your torso perpendicular to the ground, lower yourself until your left thigh is almost parallel to the floor. Your right leg should be bent at almost 90 degrees.

Action: Jump up and scissor your legs so your right leg is in front and your left leg is behind.

Land with both knees bent and your weight on the heel of your front foot and the ball of your back foot.

Repeat on the opposite side to complete 1 rep. Repeat the sequence for the designated number of repetitions.

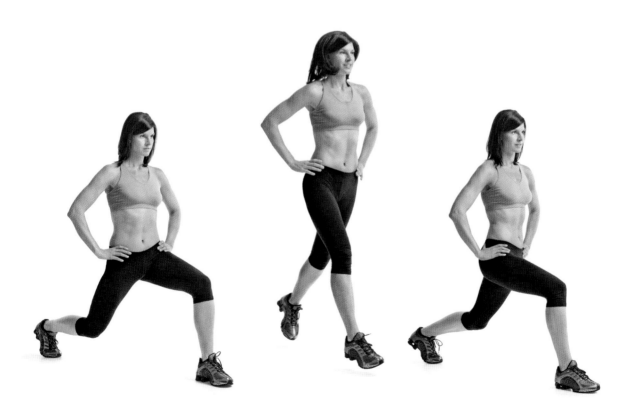

Lateral Lunge Reaches

Start: Stand tall with your feet together and arms reaching skyward.

Action: Step out with your right foot into a lunge and reach your hands past your knee toward the floor. Push off your right foot to return to the start position to complete 1 rep, then repeat on your left side.

Continue alternating sides for the designated number of repetitions.

Note: Make sure to always keep your front knee over the ankle of your front foot to avoid injury.

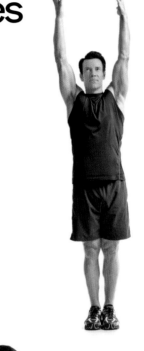

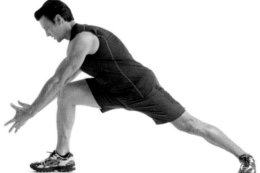

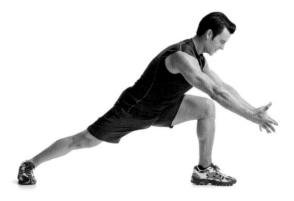

Jack-in-the-Box Jump Squats

Start: Place your feet about shoulder-width apart. Lower your hips into a squat until your thighs are almost parallel to the floor. Cross your arms in front of you.

Action: Jump explosively in the air and spread your arms and legs wide.

Land with your feet together and quickly lower yourself back to the start position.

Repeat for the designated number of repetitions.

Trainer's Tip: Land softly on the balls of your feet for every rep, with your heels barely touching the floor. Each repetition begins with a momentary pause at the lowered start position.

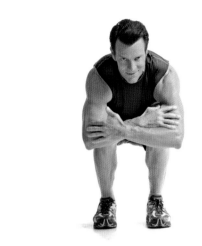

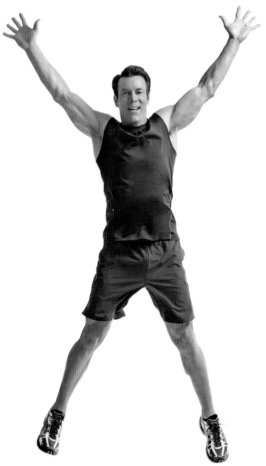

Plyometric Squats

Start: Begin with your feet in a narrow stance. Keep your arms at your sides.

Action: Bend your knees to lower yourself into a squat position.

Jump into the air, raising your arms above your head.

Land with your feet back in a narrow stance and go right back into a squat. Repeat for the designated number of repetitions. Each squat counts as 1 repetition.

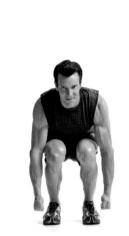
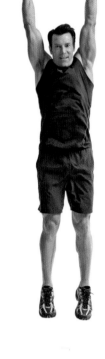

Wide-Feet Plyometric Squat Variation:
Perform the above move, but with your legs positioned more than shoulder-width apart. Then jump upward, maintaining the wide stance, and bring your hands overhead.

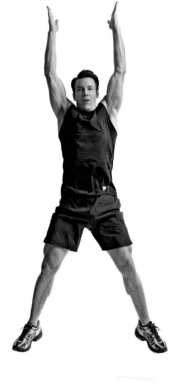
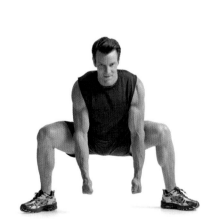

Jump Knee Tucks/Low Squat Hops

Start: Stand with your feet about 12 inches apart. Hold your arms out in front of your chest, parallel to the floor and palms facing down.

Action: Jump up as high as you can, bringing your legs as close to your buttocks as possible.

Land on the floor with your knees bent and in a low squat. Repeat for the designated number of repetitions.

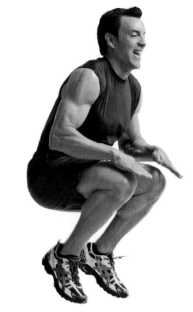

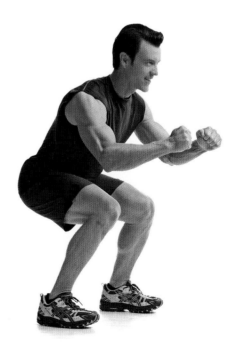

Super Cardio Moves

Jumping Jacks

Start: Stand with your feet together and arms at your sides. Keep your core engaged (tightened) to pull your pelvis forward and take the curve out of your lower back.

Action: Bend your knees and jump, moving your feet apart until they are more than shoulder-width apart. At the same time, raise your arms above your head.

When you land, you should be on the balls of your feet. Keep your knees bent while you jump again, bringing your feet together and your arms back to your sides. At the end of the movement, your weight should be on your heels. Repeat the sequence for the designated number of repetitions.

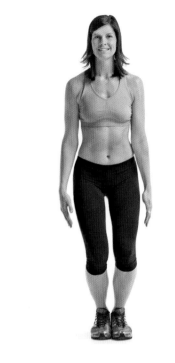

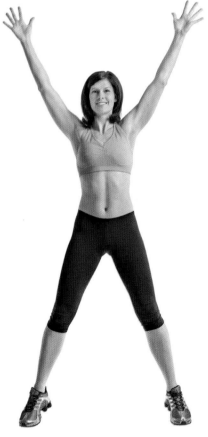

Step Jacks

Start: This is a modified version of the standard jumping jack. Begin with your feet a few inches apart and your hands at your sides.

Action: Step with your right foot out to your right side while raising your arms.

Return to the start position, then repeat the move on your left side to complete 1 rep. Continue alternating to each side for the designated number of repetitions.

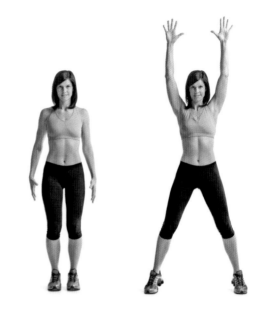

Wacky Jacks

Start: Stand with your feet slightly more than shoulder-width apart, your arms raised, and your upper arms parallel to the floor.

Action: Lift your right leg out to the side, while simultaneously bending at the waist to your right. Your right elbow should almost touch your right thigh.

Repeat on the left side.

Continue moving swiftly from side to side (this is a dynamic, fast-paced movement) for the designated number of repetitions.

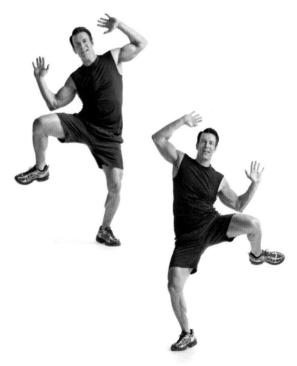

High Knee Run

Start: Stand with your feet together and arms bent at your sides.

Action: Alternating legs, begin stepping, raising your knees high with each step. As you step, pull your opposite arm up and your other arm down toward your rib cage. Continue alternating legs for the designated number of repetitions.

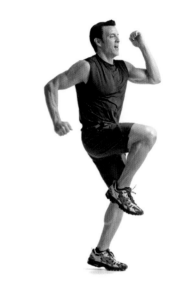

Steam Engine

Start: Stand with your feet slightly more than shoulder-width apart and your fingers interlaced behind your head, making sure to keep your elbows back.

Action: Raise your left knee diagonally up across your body as you turn your torso to touch that knee with your right elbow.

Return to the start position, and quickly repeat with the other leg to complete 1 rep.

Try to keep your head and chest up throughout the movement, and rather than leaning forward, really try to bring your knee toward your elbow. Repeat for the designated number of repetitions.

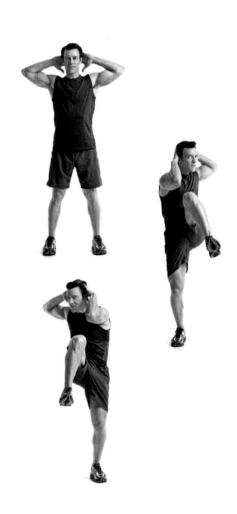

Steam Engine Kicks

Start: Stand with your feet slightly more than shoulder-width apart and your fingers interlaced behind your head, making sure to keep your elbows back.

Action: Raise your right knee diagonally up across your body as you turn your torso to touch your right knee with your left elbow. As your elbow and knee make contact, extend your leg, and then quickly return it to a bent position.

Return to the start position, and quickly repeat with the other leg to complete 1 rep.

Try to keep your head and chest up throughout the movement, and rather than leaning forward, really try to bring your knee toward your elbow. Repeat for the designated number of repetitions.

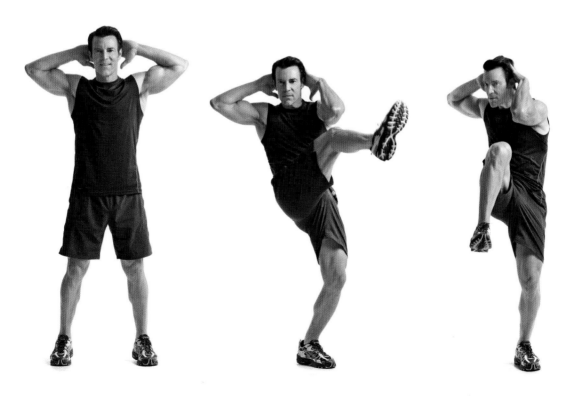

Lunge and Catch

Start: Stand with your feet much more than shoulder-width apart and your hands extended far out in front of you to the left, as if you're catching a ball.

Action: Keeping your legs wide, turn and pivot to the opposite side. Repeat back and forth as quickly as possible for the designated number of repetitions.

Note: Be sure to pivot on the balls of your feet to avoid injury. The further you reach and the deeper you lunge the better.

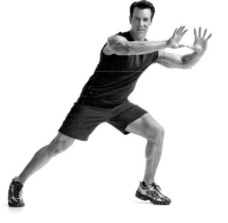
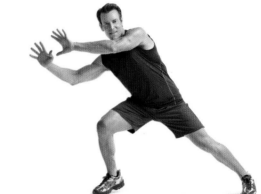

Squat Walk

Start: Stand in a squat position with your legs more than shoulder-width apart and your right foot forward, left foot back, and hands in the fighter's stance (be sure to keep your butt down and your head and chest up).

Action: Maintaining the low squat position, walk forward 4 steps, then backward 4 steps to complete 1 rep. Repeat the sequence for the designated number of repetitions.

Trainer's Tip: Find a depth that works for you to protect your knees.

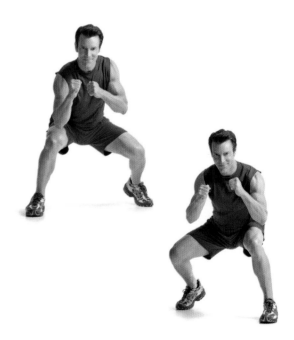

Lateral Shuffle

Start: Stand with your feet about shoulder-width apart, with your arms out in front of your chest.

Action: With your left leg leading, shuffle to the left 4 times.

Repeat the move to the right side to complete 1 rep. Repeat the sequence for the designated number of repetitions.

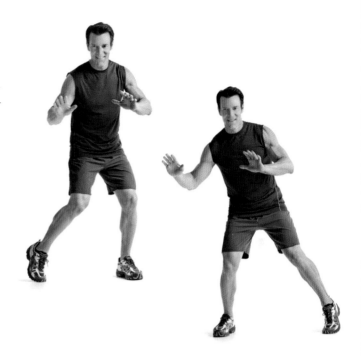

Press Jacks

Start: Stand with your feet together. Bend your elbows so that your fists are just in front of and below your chin.

Action: Jump both legs out to the sides while simultaneously bringing your arms overhead. Repeat for the designated number of repetitions.

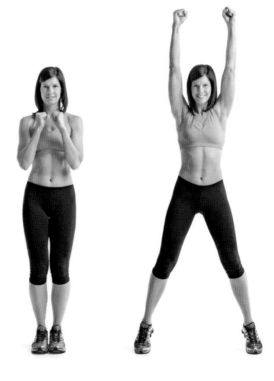

Runner's Lunge/Knee Pulls

Start: Lunge forward on your left leg. Extend your right leg behind you. Lean forward with your hands clasped in front of your chest.

Action: Bring your right leg forward to a bent-knee position. Crunch your torso down toward your right knee.

Repeat for the designed number of repetitions, then switch legs and repeat on the opposite side

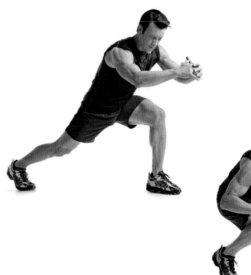
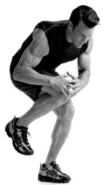

Pivot Twist

Start: Stand with your feet slightly more than shoulder-width apart. Your arms should be raised with your upper arms parallel to the floor and elbows out. Clench your fists and keep your hands close together.

Action: Twist sharply to the right while pivoting on the balls of both feet. Quickly repeat in the opposite direction, alternating back and forth as fast as possible for the designated number of repetitions. (The faster you twist and turn, the more you'll feel this in your core.)

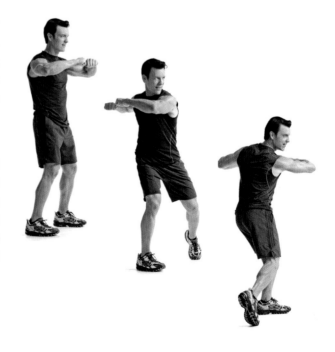

Fast Feet Football Drill

Start: Begin in a 3-point stance (deep squat, right foot forward, left foot back, right-hand fingertips on the floor).

Action: Spring up and maintain a medium squat position with your hands out in front of you as you run in place as fast as possible (with your feet barely leaving the ground) for about 5 seconds, then drop back down into a 3-point stance.

Quickly repeat the sequence for the designated number of repetitions.

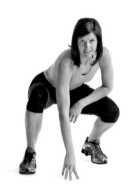

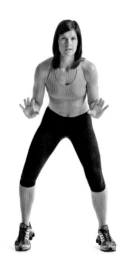

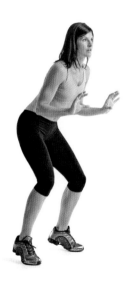

Sprint Squats

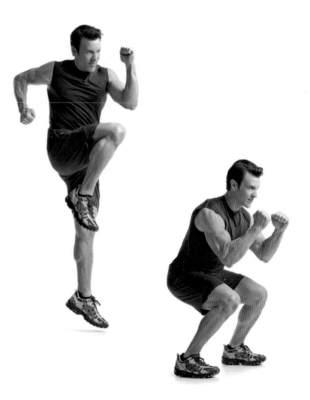

Start: Stand there getting your mind right.

Action: Sprint in place with high knees for 8 steps, then drop into a squat position with your feet slightly more than shoulder-width apart and perform 4 squats at medium pace with your hands in the fighter's stance.

Repeat the sequence for the designated number of repetitions.

Standing Speed Climbers

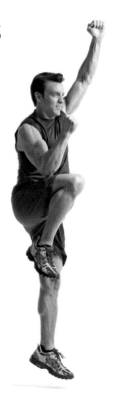

Start: Begin with your left leg straight and your left arm extended straight over your heard, and your right leg bent with the knee up and your right elbow close to your right thigh.

Action: Run in place with high knees as fast as possible while alternating your arms up and down for the designated number of repetitions.

Note: At high-knee position, the raised knee and same-side elbow should come close to touching.

Burpee Sprints

Start: Stand there getting your mind right . . . again.

Action: Quickly drop into the top of a pushup position, kicking your legs back and keeping your feet about shoulder-width apart. Then quickly jump your feet up to your hands, stand up, and immediately resume sprinting for 8 steps.

Repeat the sequence for the designated number of repetitions.

Trainer's Tip: To make this move more intense, add a pushup. If this move is too intense, you can modify it by stepping one leg back at a time, then one leg up at a time.

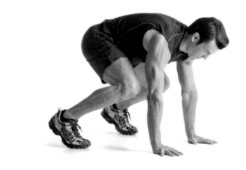

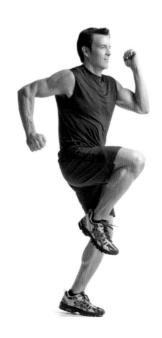

Briggs Ram

Start:
Stand with your feet slightly more than shoulder-width apart. Place your arms at your sides, slightly in front of your body, with your elbows slightly bent. Make your hands into fists (imagine holding a 40-pound steel ram, a.k.a. the master key that law enforcement uses for any and all doors).

Action:
Shift your weight to your right foot while swinging your arms across your body and upward to the right (imagine loading up to swing the ram at a door). Then shift your weight to your left foot and forcefully swing your arms across your body to the left (imagine hitting the door).

Then reverse direction and repeat the move on the other side to complete 1 rep. Continue to repeat the sequence for the designated number of repetitions.

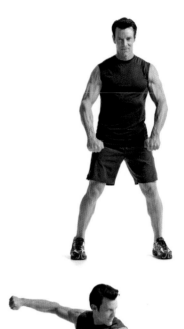

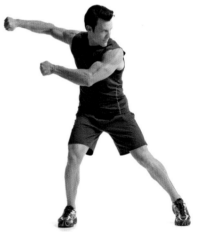

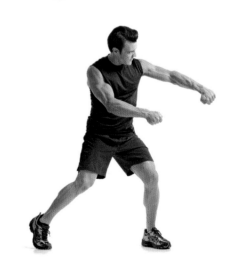

Walking Is Not Enough!

Human beings walk to get around, not to lose weight. Up until the last 30 or 40 years, most people in this country and around the world were relatively thin and fit. Most of us didn't eat processed foods loaded with fat, sugar, and salt, nor did we sit in front of screens all day and night. We walked and played and ate real food. But our lives have changed dramatically over the last 25 years. And in the process, the obesity rate has skyrocketed. A lot of people say they walk as a form of exercise—and while any activity is good activity, obesity is not a problem that's going to be solved by walking alone. The issue is and has always been "calories in versus calories out." Walking is certainly better than doing nothing, but from my experience it's not enough if you're looking for dramatic metabolic and physical changes. If you want head-over-heels dramatic change in your health and well-being, you have to do a variety of cardiovascular plus interval exercises, such as the moves I'm suggesting here.

As for jogging and running, if you love it, do it, but make sure you don't overdo it. Your hips, back, knees, and ankles will let you know soon enough that you're doing more damage than good. Research shows that young bodies can handle more, while older (you know who you are) can't. I'm 52 and even though I'm in great shape, a 15-mile run destroys me. I can handle a 5- to 6-mile jog/run at a 7½- to 8½-mile pace. I'm in my target heart rate for most of it, and it's not tearing up my joints and connective tissue. Start out by doing 20 minutes and progress from there. Warm up properly, ease into the run for the first 5 to 8 minutes, and always—I mean always—wear a heart rate monitor. Do not make running and jogging the sole cardio you do but, rather, one part of your overall heart, lung, and leg fitness program.

Tony's Motivators: Fast Change Is Proactive Change

Tiptoeing your way to dramatic change can work for some people, but I believe that sometimes you need to clean house completely to prepare yourself for life-altering, long-term change. If you went around your house right now and collected all of the crap that's been sitting around, unused, for years—and then threw it out or gave it away—you'd feel phenomenal. You must apply the same principle to your lifestyle. Let go of familiar and safe behaviors that don't work and adapt (and stick with) new, unfamiliar, challenging activities to create a better life. You can't hold on and let go at the same time. You can't work out and eat junk food. You can't work out in the morning and get drunk after work. Life is frightfully short, and I'd hate to see anyone miss out on the incredible opportunities available to all of us. We're all capable. We're all deserving. Write down all the things in your life that aren't working. Then make a list of the things you plan on doing to make your life better. Be proactive, not passive! Let go and get going.

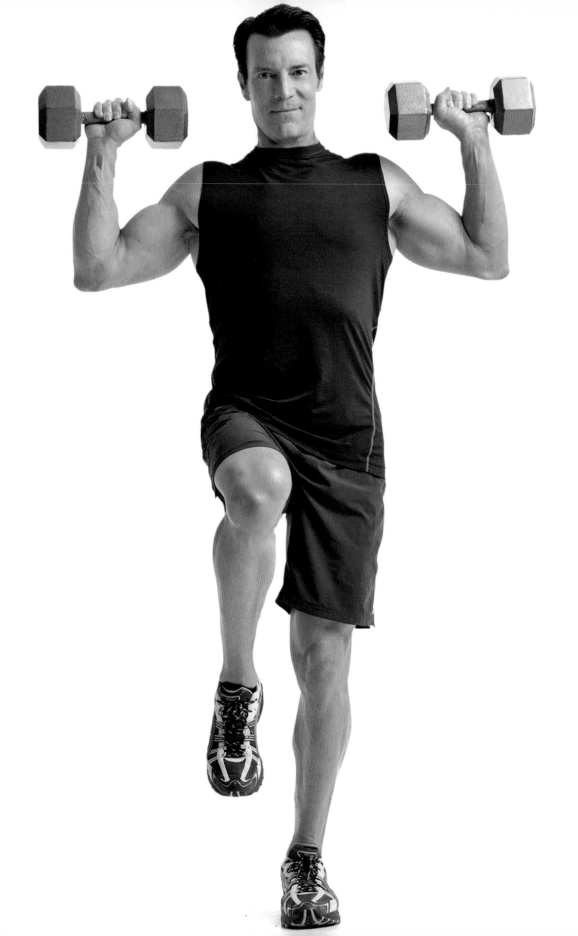

Upper Body Blasters

Your upper body plays a front-and-center role in just about any activity you can think of, from golf to volleyball to toting groceries to your car. A strong, sculpted upper body will also give you better posture, enabling you to pull your shoulders back, preventing a hunched-over posture, a protruding belly, and even nasty back and neck pain. And guys—a buff upper body adds width to your figure and makes your waist appear smaller. Yet many people neglect their upper body in order to spend time on their thighs, glutes, abs, and other problem spots.

Nature has doled out strength somewhat unevenly between the genders. Women generally have strong legs and hips, equal to and sometimes stronger than most men. That's great news for jumping, running, kicking, and so forth. Unfortunately, once we move above the waistline, men tend to be considerably stronger in a pound-for-pound comparison—in other words, in the back, arms, chest, and abs. This leaves many women at a disadvantage when it comes to upper body strength. The good news is that much of this gap can be bridged through smart training.

So, I'll take you through a whole catalog of exercises that do three things at once. First, they help strengthen your upper back and shoulders to create that sculpted V shape. Second, you'll learn moves designed to strengthen the rhomboids in your back and help improve posture. Third, I will show you chest exercises that will not only give you strength for sports and everyday activities but change your appearance as well.

Robert is a real-life example of how effective these exercises can be. I met Robert last year at one of my fitness camps. He told me that one summer he tried to squeeze into a pair of shorts and the buttons popped off! (Know the feeling?) It was a huge wake-up call for him. Robert got serious and started using P90X. After losing 20 pounds, he was able to fit into those shorts with no problem. But what he really dug was how much more sculpted his upper body had become. "No more man boobs," he told me, pulling up his shirt. "I can now see my abs!" Robert added that his upper body strength improved his bowling. He has been able to increase his ball speed, and this has boosted his average by more than 10 pins.

Fair warning: I love pushups—for several reasons. First, pushups work so many parts of the body at the same time: chest, triceps, biceps, shoulders, and core. When a lot of muscle groups operate in concert, it pushes your resistance-training calorie burn from about 6 per minute to upwards of 10 calories per minute. For another, pushups help injury-proof your muscles and improve performance. And while they're defining and refining your body, pushups are also honing skills like balance, posture, and core strength.

In addition to the standard and familiar upper body exercises, I have so many variations for you here that it will make your head spin (and your body strong and sculpted). And don't worry. Everyone can do some version of these moves. This is why my programs have helped tens of thousands of people who have never succeeded before—they work for all fitness levels. Sound good? Let's get going.

Standard Pushups

Focus: **Chest, triceps, and core**

Start: Begin by starting at the top of a pushup. Your hands should be on the floor, slightly wider than shoulder-width apart and aligned with your chest muscles. Engage your butt and belly to create a straight line from your head to your heels. Keep your feet slightly apart.

Action: Bend your arms and lower your body toward the floor, keeping your butt and core engaged. Push yourself back up to the start position and repeat for the designated number of repetitions while maintaining perfect form.

Trainer's Tip: Try to straighten your arms at the top of every rep and lower your body as close to the floor as possible based on your fitness level.

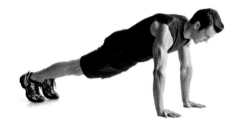

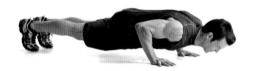

Modified Pushups

Focus: **Chest, triceps, and core**

Start: Assume the start position described above, then drop your knees to the floor and raise your feet (do not cross your ankles).

Action: Slowly bend your arms and lower your body toward the floor as close as you can based on your fitness level. Then push yourself back up to the start position and repeat for the designated number of repetitions while maintaining perfect form.

Trainer's Tip: Avoid butt rise and slack by making sure you contract the muscles of your butt and belly.

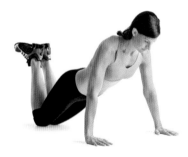

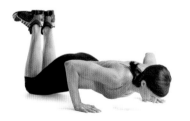

Wide-Hand Pushups
Focus: **Chest and triceps**

Start: Assume a pushup position as follows: your feet together, back straight, arms straight, and hands 2 to 3 feet apart.

Action: Bend your arms and slowly lower yourself to the floor. Lower your chest until it almost reaches the floor.

Straighten your arms and repeat for the designated number of repetitions.

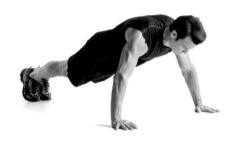

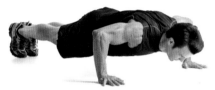

Wide-Hand and Leg Pushups
Focus: **Chest and triceps**

Start: Assume a pushup position as follows: your feet slightly more than shoulder-width apart, hands 2 to 3 feet apart.

Action: Bend your arms and slowly lower yourself to the floor. Lower your chest until it almost reaches the floor.

Straighten your arms and repeat for the designated number of repetitions.

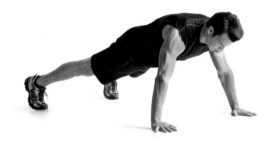

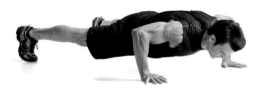

Rami Plyo Pushups
Focus: **Entire upper body**

Start: Assume a pushup position (see page 127), with your feet and hands slightly more than shoulder-width apart.

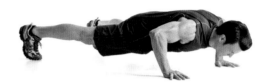

Action: Press up and literally jump off the floor while maintaining the pushup position. Repeat for the designated number of repetitions.

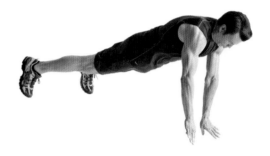

Sphinx Pushups
Focus: **Chest and triceps**

Start: Assume a pushup position as follows: your feet together and forearms and palms on the floor, with your elbows bent.

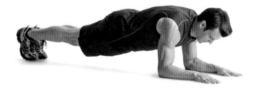

Action: Perform the pushups in the normal manner: Straighten your arms and push your body up. Slowly lower yourself until your chest almost reaches the floor.

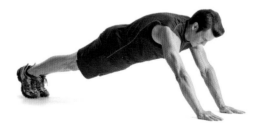

Straighten your arms and repeat for the designated number of repetitions.

Chuck-Ups
Focus: **Chest, shoulders, and triceps**

Start: Assume a pushup position with your feet together and your fingers pointed outward from your body.

Action: Lower your body until your chest is a few inches from the floor, then hold for a slow 2 count. Push yourself back up to the start position and repeat the sequence for the designated number of repetitions.

Next, rotate your fingers inward (facing each other) and repeat the above sequence for the designated number of repetitions.

Then stack your hands on top of each other and repeat the above sequence for the designated number of repetitions.

Trainer's Tip: In the first sequence, be sure to keep your elbows close to your sides. In the second, your elbows should point out away from your body. In the third, your elbows should point out at an angle, slightly away from your sides.

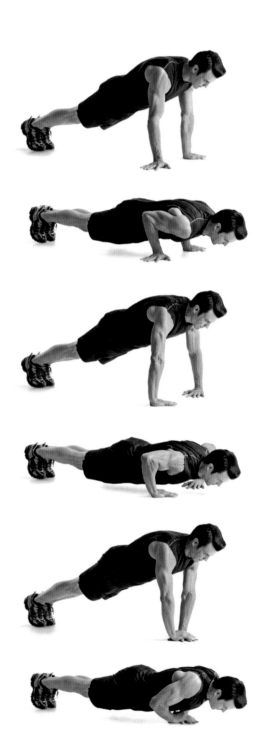

Standing Shoulder Presses
Focus: **Shoulders**

Start: Stand with your feet about shoulder-width apart and offset (one foot forward, one foot back). Grasp a dumbbell in each hand and hold them just above shoulder level, palms facing forward.

Action: Press your arms overhead, rotating your palms inward, and straighten your arms at the top of the movement. Return your arms to the start position and repeat for the designated number of repetitions.

Advanced Version: Follow the same instructions, but perform the exercise while balancing on one foot. Switch your standing leg for each set.

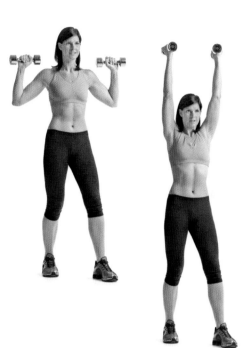

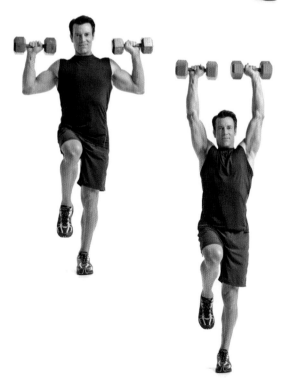

One-Foot Curl and Presses
Focus: Shoulders and arms

Start: Stand on one foot, holding a dumbbell in each hand.

Action: Perform a standard biceps curl. At the top of the movement, rotate your palms forward and press the dumbbells overhead.

Lower the dumbbells and repeat for the designated number of repetitions.

Trainer's Tip: Switch your standing leg for each set.

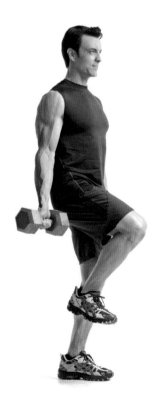
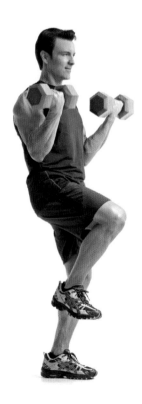
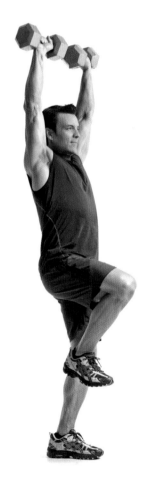

Upright Row Y-Presses
Focus: **Shoulders**

Start: Begin with your feet shoulder-width apart and offset with one foot slightly behind the other (to protect your lower back throughout the motion). Hold a dumbbell in each hand, arms hanging in front of your body and palms facing you.

Action: Engage your core, keep your chest tall, and pull the dumbbells to collarbone level while keeping your elbows high. Then rotate the dumbbells just above shoulder height (palms facing out, elbows down) and perform a shoulder press with your hands wide at the top.

Perform the movement in reverse and repeat for the designated number of repetitions.

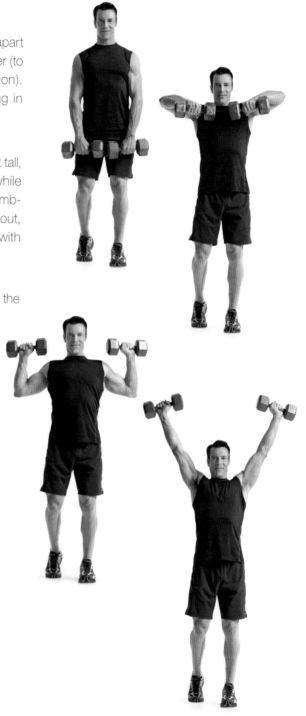

Standing Swimmer's Presses
Focus: **Shoulders and arms**

Start: Stand with your feet slightly more than shoulder-width apart, with one foot slightly behind the other. Grasp a dumbbell in each hand.

Action: Lift the dumbbells as you would for a biceps curl, so the dumbbells are resting near your chest with your palms facing toward you.

Push the dumbbells toward the ceiling. As you lift the dumbbells, rotate your palms so they face away from your body. Then fully extend your arms upward.

Lower the dumbbells back and reverse the twisting action so your palms are facing your body once again.

Repeat for the designated number of repetitions.

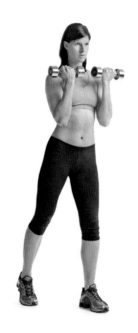

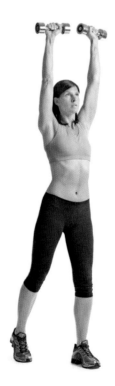

Straight-Arm Posterior Delt Flies

Focus: **Shoulders and upper back**

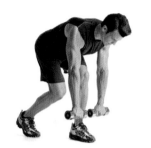

Start: Bend forward at the waist so that your torso is nearly parallel to the floor. Place one foot slightly behind the other. Grasp a pair of dumbbells in an overhand grip, with your palms facing toward your body. Extend your arms toward the floor.

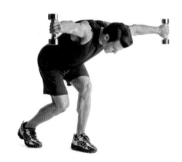

Action: Raise your arms out to your sides, pointing the ends of the dumbbells toward the ceiling. Squeeze your back muscles in the top position. Slowly lower to the start position. Repeat for the designated number of repetitions.

Bent-Over Rows

Focus: **Upper back, lower back, and rear shoulders**

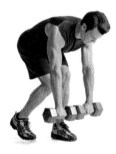

Start: Stand with your feet shoulder-width apart, with one foot slightly behind the other. Bend forward at the waist so that your torso is nearly parallel to the floor. Grasp a dumbbell in each hand and hold them extended down in front of you.

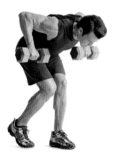

Action: Bend your elbows and pull the dumbbells straight up, nearly to your armpits. Squeeze your back muscles in the top position. Slowly lower to the start position. Repeat for the designated number of repetitions.

Shoulder Flies with Band
Focus: **Shoulders**

Start: Holding the handles of a resistance band, stand on the center of the band with your left foot. Separate your feet wide with your right foot offset and behind your left.

Action: Raise your arms laterally, keeping them bent (about 90 degrees at the top), and keep your forearms parallel to the floor at the top of the movement.

Return to the start position and repeat for the designated number of repetitions.

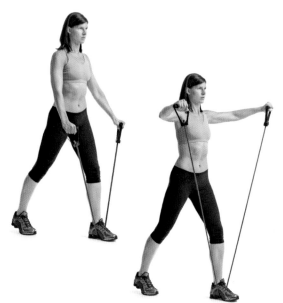

Shoulder Flies on One Foot
Focus: **Shoulders, core, and balance**

Start: Hold a dumbbell in each hand, palms facing inward. Stand on one leg.

Action: Raise your arms laterally and begin to bend and raise your elbows so your forearms are parallel to the floor at the top of the motion.

Return to the start position and repeat for the designated number of repetitions.

Trainer's Tip: Switch your standing leg for each set.

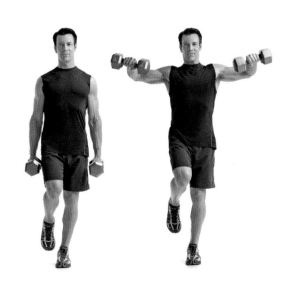

One-Foot Rear Delt Flies with Band

Focus: **Rear shoulders and back**

Start: Make a small loop with a resistance band on the floor and stand on the loop with your left foot. Holding the handles, raise your right foot off the floor, keeping your back flat and core engaged as you lean slightly forward.

Action: Pull the band up and out away from your body, bending your elbows toward the ceiling. When your upper arms are parallel to the floor, lower the band back to the start position in a slow, controlled movement.

Repeat for the designated number of repetitions.

Trainer's Tip: Switch your standing leg for each set.

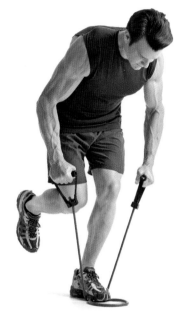

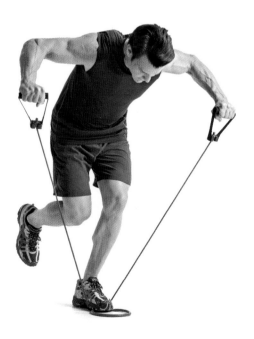

Upright Rows
Focus: Upper back and arms

Start: Stand with your feet about shoulder-width apart. Place one foot slightly behind the other. Grasp a pair of dumbbells and hold your arms straight down, palms facing your thighs.

Action: Bend your elbows and pull the dumbbells up to just under your chin. Your elbows will naturally flare out and up at the top of the movement. Lower to the start position and repeat for the designated number of repetitions.

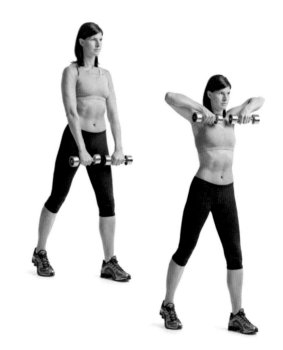

Lawnmowers
Focus: Back

Start: Step forward on your left foot with your right leg extended behind you. Your torso should be at a slight forward-leaning angle. Hold a dumbbell in your right hand with your arm extended straight to the floor.

Action: Pull the weight up to your waist (as if you're starting a lawnmower). Return to the start position in a slow and controlled movement, and repeat for the designated number of repetitions. Switch legs and hands and repeat on the opposite side.

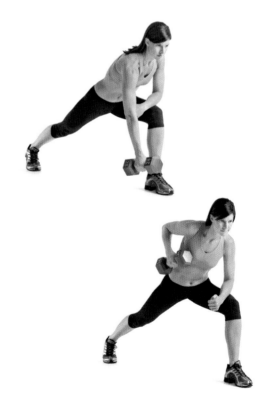

Pullups
Focus: **Back and shoulders**

Start: Place your hands on the bar with an over-hand grip and slightly more than shoulder-width apart.

Action: Pull your body up until your chin clears the bar, then lower yourself to the start position in a slow, controlled movement. Repeat for the designated number of repetitions based on your fitness level.

Trainer's Tip: Do your best to maintain perfect form by avoiding the recruitment of your lower body in a kicking movement (a.k.a. "kipping" or "body English") to assist you in getting your chin over the bar.

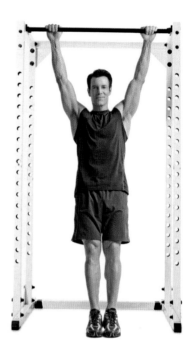

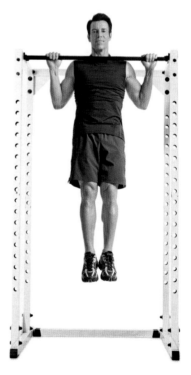

Chair-Assist Pullup Modification
Focus: Back and shoulders

Start: Place your hands on the bar with an overhand grip and slightly more than shoulder-width apart. Place one of your feet on the chair to provide extra support.

Action: Pull your body up to the bar and attempt to get your chin over the bar. Keep your foot on the chair for needed leverage. Lower your body and repeat for the designated number of repetitions (maintaining good form).

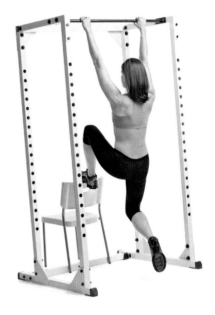

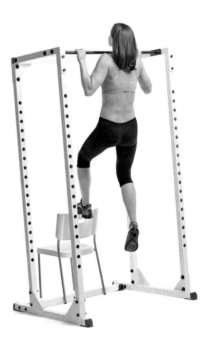

Switch-Grip Pullups
Focus: Back, shoulders, and biceps

Start: Place your hands on the bar with an overhand grip and slightly more than shoulder-width apart. Keep your feet together. Note: If you are using a door-mounted pullup bar, you will need to bend your knees.

Action: Perform 2 pullups, then place your feet on the floor momentarily and switch to an underhand grip (chinup position). Perform 2 chinups, then transition back to an overhand grip.

Continue the sequence for the designated number of repetitions.

Advanced Switch-Grip Pullups:
Perform the above sequence without placing your feet on the floor when you switch grip positions. Note: A door-mounted pullup bar would not be safe to use for this movement.

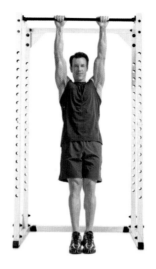
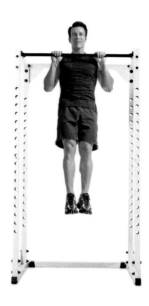
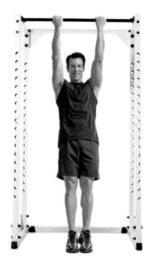
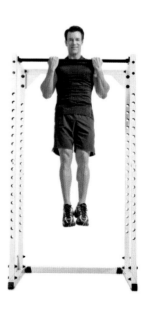

Wide-to-Narrow Pullups
Focus: **Back and biceps**

Start: Place your hands on the bar more than shoulder-width apart with your palms facing away from your body. Extend your legs to the sides.

Action: Perform a pullup as described on page 139. However, after 1 wide-grip pullup, move your legs and hands together and perform 1 close-grip pullup. Return to the start position and repeat.

Alternate in this fashion for the designated number of repetitions.

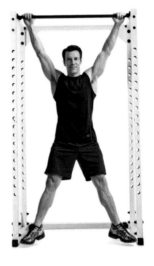
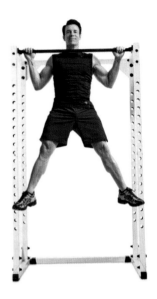
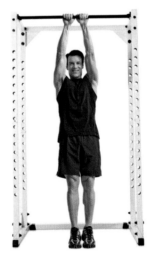
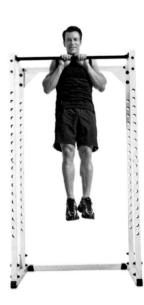

Wide-Hand Pullups

Focus: **Back, biceps, and core**

Start:
Place your hands on the bar about shoulder-width apart with your palms facing away from your body.

Action:
Bend your elbows and pull your body straight up so that your chin is over the bar. Lower your body to the start position. Repeat for the designated number of repetitions.

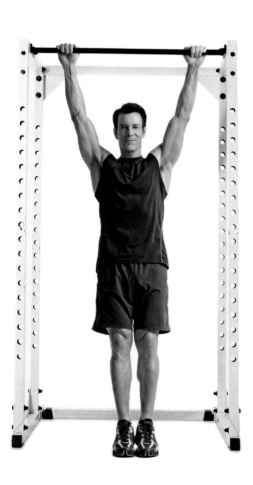

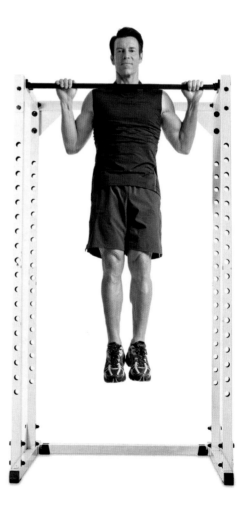

Levers

Focus: **Back, shoulders, triceps, core . . . everything!**

Start: Place your hands on the bar slightly more than shoulder-width apart with your palms facing away from your body.

Action: Unlike a traditional pullup, straighten your arms as you push your upper body away (not down) from the bar as you lever your lower body into a horizontal position. Then begin to bend your elbows to return to the top of a pullup position as you lever your body back to the vertical start position.

Repeat for the designated number of repetitions.

Note: This advanced gymnastic pullup move requires that you lock every muscle in your core and lower body. It's imperative that you *do not* bend at your waist or knees.

Trainer's Tip: This move requires time, patience, and practice.

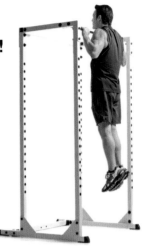

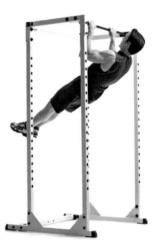

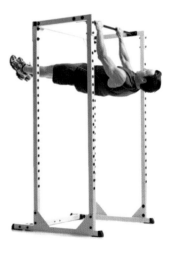

Chinups
Focus: **Back and biceps**

Start: Place your hands on the bar in an underhand grip position and about shoulder-width apart.

Action: Pull your chin up past the bar, then lower yourself in a slow and controlled movement to the start position. Repeat for the designated number of repetitions.

Trainer's Tip: With any chinup or pullup, it's always important to focus on using a full range of motion with your shoulders still engaged at the bottom position of the movement.

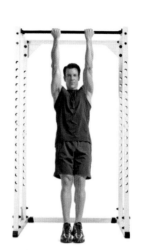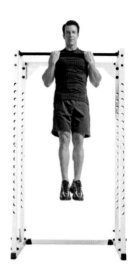

Knee-Up Chinups
Focus: **Back, biceps, and core**

Start: Place your hands on the bar in an underhand grip position and about shoulder-width apart. Keep your feet together and bend your knees so that your thighs are parallel to the floor.

Action: Perform a chinup while keeping your legs in the start position. Repeat for the designated number of repetitions.

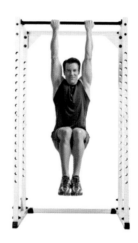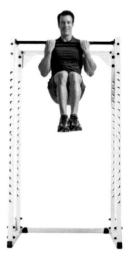

Two-Ball Pike Presses
Focus: Shoulders, triceps, and core

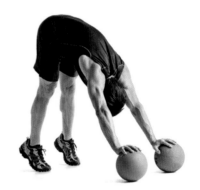

Start: Place two medicine balls on the floor slightly more than shoulder-width apart. Get into a standard pushup position with each hand on top of a medicine ball. Walk your feet to your hands until your body is in the shape of a capital A. Raise your heels off the floor so you are on the balls of your feet and straighten your arms while keeping your core engaged.

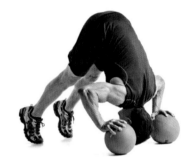

Action: Bend your arms and lower the crown of your head to about 1 inch from the floor. Straighten your arms to return to the start position and repeat for the designated number of repetitions while maintaining good form.

Heavy Pants
Focus: Upper back

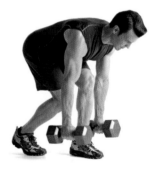

Start: Stand with your feet about shoulder-width apart, one foot slightly behind the other. Hold a dumbbell in each hand. Bend forward at your waist and, while keeping your back flat, straighten your arms down with the dumbbells at each side of your front ankle.

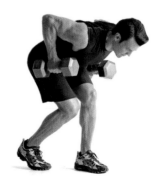

Action: Bending your elbows, pull the dumbbells straight up toward your hips and waist. Return to the start position in a slow and controlled movement and repeat for the designated number of repetitions.

Trainer's Tip: Maintain a flat back and engage your core throughout the movement to avoid lower back injury. Lower weight and higher repetitions are recommended for this exercise.

Tony's Motivators: A Mobile Workout

The exercises and workouts you're learning in this book are entirely mobile—you can do them anywhere, anytime, even when you're traveling. In fact, coincidentally enough, just as this book was headed to print I received an e-mail from a travel writer, who wrote:

"My job is designed to make me fat. If my colleagues and I aren't eating chicken parm on an airplane, we're eating candy and doughnuts while waiting for an airplane. If we're not eating a ridiculous, seven-course meal at some fancy restaurant, we're eating a cheeseburger and fries at a train station. We'll follow 34-hour flights (connecting at some airport, with more candy and doughnuts) with a 10-hour drive (more candy! more doughnuts!) and then maybe 2 days of food poisoning in southeast Asia. It's a great job but a terrible lifestyle.

"Thankfully, I can work out on the road. The best thing for me about your workouts is that they're completely mobile. I've done them everywhere from Jodhpur, India, to Buenos Aires, Argentina, in dozens of hotel gyms and city parks. I was a fat kid, doing aerobics-only routines at 11 years old and trying to get by on a cup of watered-down chicken noodle soup for meals. That didn't work. But your workouts do. At 35, I'm stronger and fitter than I've ever been—and that includes being able to complete two marathons.

"So tell your readers not to let travel derail their workouts! All you need is some packable work-out gear like resistance bands, maybe some light dumbbells, and your own body weight. There's no excuse to get out of shape while on the road."

If a professional traveler can find a way to exercise on the road, so can you. When you know you're going to be away from home for a while, plan for your workouts. Pack your gym clothes and shoes, bring along this book or a DVD, and do a few quick workouts in your hotel gym or even your hotel room. You'll be glad you did when you return home and can still manage to button your jeans.

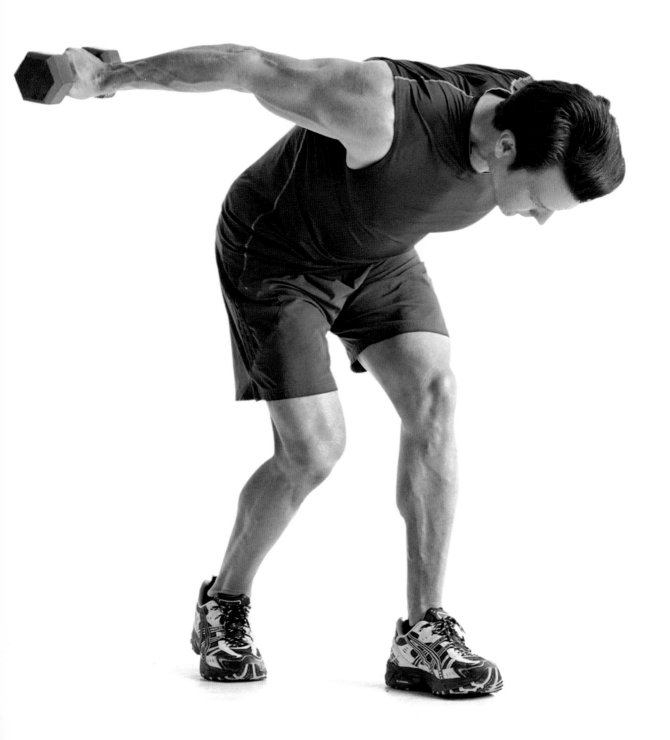

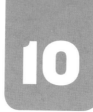

Firm Arms Fast

Have you ever found yourself sweltering under the

summer sun because you didn't want to be caught in a sleeveless top? Then I'm sure you know what it's like to long for buff arms. One of the most revealing characteristics of people who are in great shape is their sculpted arms.

Arms respond quickly to training. Unlike other parts of the body (like thighs), there's less fat to deal with, so arms are usually the first body part to "bare" the positive signs of consistent training. If you've got skinny, scrawny arms, you'll get fast results, too.

For all this to happen, the key is to incorporate variety into your arm training. Besides altering sets, reps, and resistances used, you can change it up by varying grip width (narrow, medium, wide), grip position (both pronated, both supinated, or an alternating grip), and angle of pull. Simply change one of these factors each workout. That way you'll be sure to blast lots of different muscle fibers in your arms on your way to greater tone and strength.

The exercises in this chapter focus mainly on your biceps and triceps. The biceps are the more visible muscle that gives your arm its shape—and the arm muscle everyone wants to work. Triceps, which make up two-thirds of the arm, are the upper body's version of thighs: They store ugly fat. Keeping them toned is key to battling arm bulge and wiggles that come with age and disuse. So my first rule of an arm workout is: Don't be afraid to target those triceps.

When my female clients demand more sculpted, shapely arms, I prescribe a challenging program of moves that use weights and resistance bands—and plenty of repetitions. This approach not only imparts strength and tone but also helps build stamina. And by the way, this approach works for guys, too.

For arms, I've chosen some killer moves designed with maximum results and minimum time in mind. These exercises are effective because they target each muscle and really challenge it. The efficiency part comes from the fact that many of the moves work both arms simultaneously.

By using these exercises faithfully in your prescribed routine, you can expect increased strength in 2 to 3 weeks and visible results in 3 to 4 weeks. Then it's so long, sleeves—hello, halters and tank tops!

Standing Biceps Curls
Focus: **Biceps**

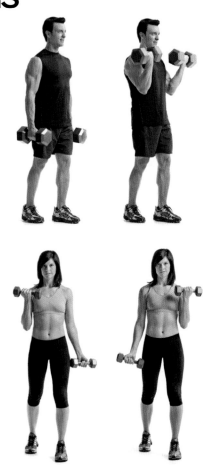

Start: Stand with your feet about shoulder-width apart, with one foot slightly behind the other. Hold a dumbbell in each hand, keeping your arms at your sides, palms facing inward.

Action: Bend your elbows and rotate your palms forward as you pull the dumbbells up toward shoulder level. Be sure to keep your elbows at your sides (do not let them move forward away from your body). Flex your biceps tightly at the top of the movement, then lower the dumbbells in a slow and controlled motion back to the start position.

Repeat for the designated number of repetitions.

Alternating Biceps Curl Variation: Perform the same move as described above, but alternate your arms, curling one arm at a time.

21s
Focus: **Biceps**

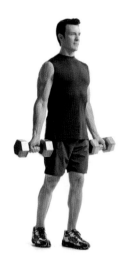

Start: Stand with your feet about a foot apart, with one foot slightly behind the other. Grasp a dumbbell in each hand and hold them at your sides, palms facing forward.

Action: There are three parts to this exercise.

Bend your elbows and start to do a curl. Lift the dumbbells until you have done half of your normal movement. In other words, instead of curling your arms all the way up to your chest, stop when your forearms are parallel to the ground. Repeat for 7 reps.

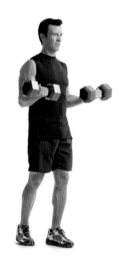

Next, do only the second half of the movement: Start with your forearms parallel to the ground and lift the dumbbells up to your chest, then back to the parallel position. Repeat for 7 reps.

Finally, perform a full curl movement. Begin with the dumbbells in the down position and do a full curl up to your chest. Repeat for 7 reps.

Bent-Over 21s Variation: Perform the exercise above with the following variation: Stand with one foot slightly behind the other, bend at the waist, and let your arms hang from the floor as you do each set of curls.

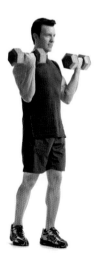

Crazy 8s
Focus: **Biceps**

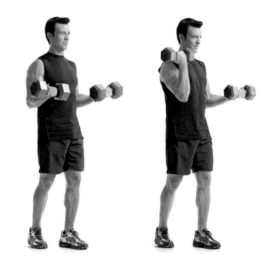

Start: Stand with your feet hip-width apart, with one foot slightly behind the other. Grasp a dumbbell in each hand. Curl both arms up to chest level.

Action: Alternate curling upward to your shoulders and downward to the chest-level position, palms facing up. Continue alternating arms until you have completed the designated number of repetitions.

In and Out Biceps Curls
Focus: **Biceps**

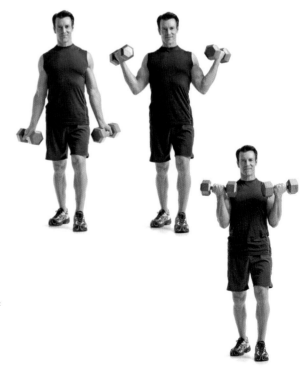

Start: Bend your knees slightly, placing one leg slightly behind the other. Keep your back straight and your shoulders relaxed. Grasp the dumbbells with your palms facing forward. Let your arms hang down by your sides with your elbows loose, not locked.

Action: For the first repetition, flare your lower arms outward while completing a curl.

Return to the start position. On the next repetition, keep your arms and elbows tight against your sides while you complete a curl.

Continue alternating for the designated number of repetitions.

Standing Double-Arm Triceps Presses

Focus: **Triceps**

Start: Stand with your feet slightly apart, with one foot slightly behind the other. Grasp one dumbbell with both hands. Bend your elbows and hold the weight behind your head. Keep your back straight and knees slightly flexed.

Action: Raise your arms overhead and lock your elbows. Return slowly to the start position. Repeat for the designated number of repetitions.

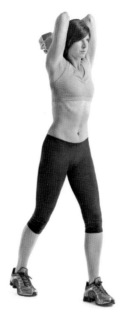

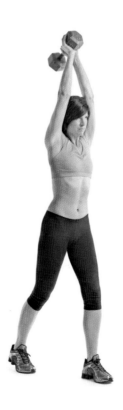

Bent-Over Switch-Grip Triceps Extensions

Focus: **Triceps**

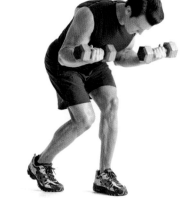

Start: Stand with your feet slightly less than shoulder-width apart, with your right foot back and your left foot forward (adjust foot position based on your balance). While holding a dumbbell in each hand with palms facing up, lean forward at the waist and, keeping your back flat and your core engaged, bend your elbows so that your forearms are parallel to the floor.

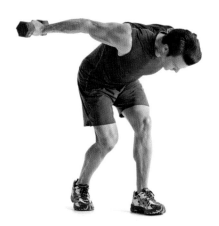

Action: While maintaining proper body position and keeping your elbows high, straighten your arms behind you. Return to the start position and flip your palms toward the floor. Straighten your arms behind you, then return to the start position.

Repeat the entire sequence for the designated number of repetitions.

Trainer's Tip: It's best to use lighter dumbbells while learning this movement.

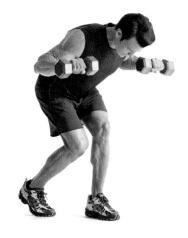

One Arm (Behind the Head) Triceps Extensions

Focus: **Triceps and shoulders**

Start: Stand with your feet slightly less than shoulder-width apart, with your right foot back and your left foot forward (adjust foot position based on your balance). Hold a dumbbell in your right hand behind your head, with your elbow pointing skyward. Place your left hand on your waist.

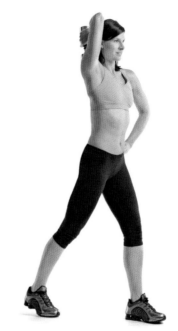

Action: Extend your right arm overhead, focusing on keeping your elbow in the start position as you straighten your arm. Lower the dumbbell to the start position and repeat for the designated number of repetitions. Switch arm and foot positions and repeat on the opposite side.

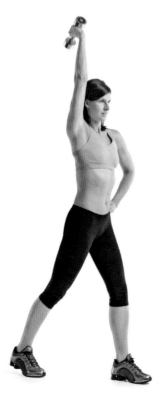

Side Tri-Rises
Focus: **Triceps, shoulders, chest, and core**

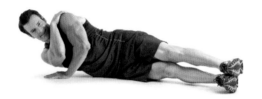

Start: Lie on your right side with your legs and feet stacked. Place your right hand on your left shoulder and your left hand on the floor under your right shoulder.

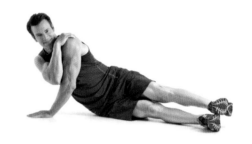

Action: Straighten your left arm (to the best of your ability), raising your upper body off the floor. Lower and repeat for the designated number of repetitions. Switch sides and repeat.

Split-Leg Side Tri-Rise
Focus: **Triceps, shoulders, chest, and core**

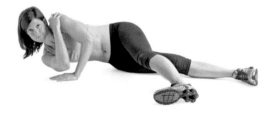

Start: Lie on your right side with your right leg in front and your left leg slightly behind.

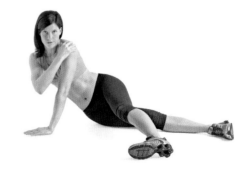

Action: Straighten your left arm (to the best of your ability), raising your upper body off the floor. Lower and repeat for the designated number of repetitions. Switch sides and repeat.

Tony's Motivators: Put on the Breaks

Sometimes you have to reevaluate your progress and take some breaks to get back on track. Here's when you might have to put on the "breaks."

Midset mini-break. Say you're working your biceps and you've mistakenly chosen a weight that's a bit too heavy. You've set a goal of 10 reps, but on rep 6 you've discovered that you're not going to make it to 10. Stop for a beat. Hold the weights down by your sides. When you're ready, continue to 10. You can also put the weights down and grab lighter ones. This technique works with almost any exercise.

Give yourself a break. Far too often I see someone trying to be a superhero during the first couple weeks of a program. This aggressive attitude can often cause stomach upset. To prevent this from happening to you, I recommend *not* trying to "push through it." Superman wasn't built in 2 weeks. He was born on an icy planet and . . . well, that's another story. Do yourself a favor and kick it down to 80 percent when you first start out.

Illness or injury breaks. If you're sick or injured, then do the right thing: Back off, back down, or modify. Hard exercise when injured or ill can be disastrous. Think long term. More often than not, taking a break is the smartest approach for lasting success.

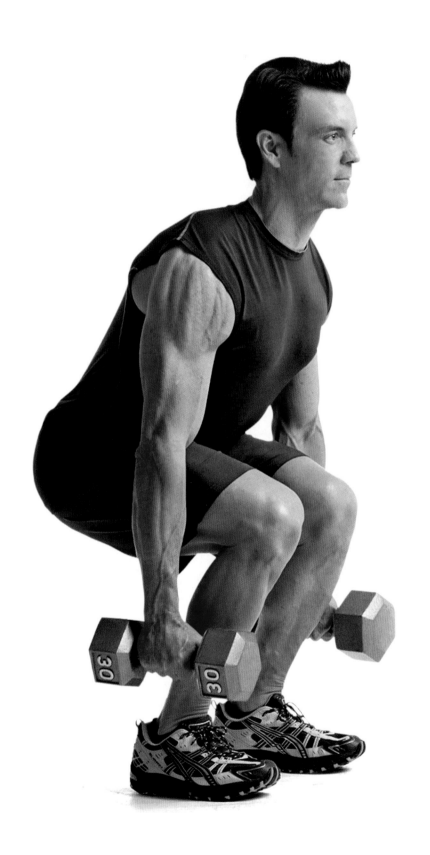

Lower Body Blitzers

Ask 20 women what they want most out of their

workouts, and at least half of them will say sleeker, shapelier, jiggle-proof thighs. And if you pose the same question to men, many of the guys will say they want more muscle to fill out their skinny legs.

Think these are impossible dreams? Think again. You can change the shape and size of your thighs, along with the rest of your lower body. You just need the right moves, variety, and consistency.

Training your lower body correctly has amazing effects on your *entire* body. Your lower body, due to its large muscle groups, is the engine that burns fat elsewhere: in your waist, butt, back, and arms. Here's how: First, you damage an expanse of muscle tissue. By working all those muscles harder than they're used to working, you make tiny tears in the muscle fibers. When your body repairs this muscle damage, its main fuel is fat. It collects particles of fat from all over your body, carries them through your blood, and uses the energy from the fat to heal the muscle.

Of course, the fat on your lower body can be notoriously stubborn to move, especially if you're a woman. Because women are designed to have children, they tend to be pear-shaped, and therefore, fat is likely to accumulate in the hips, buttocks, and inner- and outer-thigh areas. Your body is genetically programmed to deposit fat in certain areas, and the first place you put it on is generally the last place you'll take it off. It's just a tough break that the thighs are one of the most common places for women to put on extra fat. But that's not to say shaping up is hopeless.

Using lots of heavy weight may seem like the best way to whip those thighs and the rest of your lower body into shape, but a heavy workload isn't the answer. One of the techniques I recommend is high-repetition training, and for many of my lower body exercises, you don't need any equipment, just your body weight. Trust me, you'll see the results you want. Of course, there's no such thing as spot reduction. But it is possible to spot tighten, spot tone, and reshape with my methods.

If you push the envelope in terms of how many reps you do in each set, along with short rest periods between sets, you'll find that you stress your cardiovascular system immensely, as well. Also, my lower body exercises will do more than tighten, tone, and strengthen; they will also help reduce the appearance of cellulite better than any jogging, biking, or walking routine ever will.

If you're athletically inclined, the exercises you'll learn here will work wonders. Just ask Dawson Ransome, age 41, a former professional athlete. He competed as an amateur and professional road cyclist from 1990 to 1996, and he finished fourth in the U.S. National Cycling Championships in 1994. Prior to cycling, Dawson also competed in the sport of motocross and won the 1986 U.S. Amateur Motocross Championship.

After retiring from athletics in 1996, Dawson founded his own real estate company. He spent long hours sitting, and with the recent decline in the real estate market, lots of time stressing out over it. "I had no motivation to work out and wasn't interested in pedaling a bike anymore," he wrote me.

As you can guess, Dawson's former level of fitness plummeted. His once superstrong cycling legs were weak. He was 15 pounds overweight. Worried, Dawson's wife purchased P90X and encouraged him to try it with her. "First and foremost, I wanted to spend more time with her, so I participated," he said.

By the end of 90 days, a transformation had taken place, not just in his lower body strength, but elsewhere, too. I'll let Dawson tell you in his own words:

"Now I can't wait to get up and do my workout. I'm back to eating the way I know I should. My mind is better. My mood is better. I am better able to cope with daily stresses. Spiritually, I am better than I have ever been. I feel like myself again and feel better than I did when I was 20."

Consistent, high-variety, fun workouts did that for Dawson, and they can do it for you!

My Best Lower Body Move

Oh—I should mention here that as much as I like pushups, I also like squats. Years ago, I would do squats in just about every leg workout, but then I got bored with them. My waning desire to squat was an indication that my training was getting stale, and this lack of motivation translated into less-effective workouts for other muscle groups, too. Since this is the case, I knew I couldn't expect much to happen in the gains department. A change was in order! I started experimenting with different variations on the squat. What you'll learn here is how to do not only regular squats but also a dozen other versions, which appear in this chapter and Chapter 8.

One of these versions—a one-legged squat—has been shown in research to be the very best exercise for your glutes, the muscles that give shape to your buttocks. In a study at San Diego State University, researchers studied 31 women, ages 19 to 41, who performed 10 of the most commonly prescribed butt-bettering exercises while wired to a machine that measured muscle activity. The one-footed squat surpassed all the other exercises in effectiveness.[1] Because you place all of your body weight on one foot, the muscles of just one side lift your entire body. This is also an excellent balance and strengthening exercise. (Beginners may want to lightly hold on to a secure object for balance while performing it.)

The squat in all its different variations is perhaps the most effective resistance-training exercise for total-body development. It may look as if your legs are doing all of the work, but it takes a stable trunk and strong upper body to provide a foundation on which your legs can produce force.

No matter what form the squat takes, many different muscles are forced to work together. The squat involves nearly all the muscles in your thighs, your calves (for balance), and your back muscles (to keep you upright). In fact, the squat targets more than 250 muscles! This muscle orchestra also generates a serious release of muscle-growing hormones that flood your entire body. And that means muscle tone and development, plus fat burning and accelerated results.

Although the majority of my squats involve the use of your body weight only, other types of equipment can be used to boost your intensity. For example, dumbbells can be used in most cases by holding them at your sides or atop your shoulders to add the desired resistance. Resistance bands can also be effective because they allow for a little more control than their dumbbell counterpart.

Learn to love the squat, because you're going to do it a lot!

Time Efficiency

Most people I work with either hate going to the gym or have limited time, so I try to choose exercises that will get them in and out as quickly as possible. Compound moves like squats and lunges are very efficient because they get you moving in multiple directions and improve your range of motion. I think squats are more fun and effective than isolation exercises, too, because you're getting more work done in a shorter amount of time.

Targeting the Lower Body

My lower body exercises target all your major lower body muscles: the quadriceps muscles on the front of each thigh, the hamstring muscles on the rear of each thigh, the gluteal muscles (glutes) in your buttocks and hips, the abductor and adductor muscles in your inner and outer thighs, and the gastrocnemius and soleus muscles in your calves. Also involved are the iliopsoas (hip flexors), which are activated every time you bend at the hips (as in a squat), and other hip-rotator muscles that stabilize your pelvis.

Lower Body Exercises

Shoulder-Width Squats
Focus: **Thighs and buttocks**

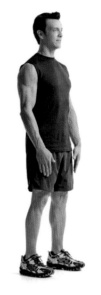

Start: Stand tall with your feet shoulder-width apart and your arms relaxed at your sides.

Action: Bend at your knees, placing your weight on your heels, and lower your thighs until they are no lower than parallel to the floor. Raise your arms out in front of you for balance while lowering (this also helps you keep your head and chest up and buttocks down at the bottom of the movement). Return to the start position and repeat for the designated number of repetitions.

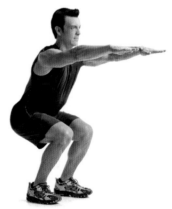

Advanced Version: For an extra challenge, try this exercise while holding a dumbbell in each hand at your sides.

Trainer's Tip: It's critical that this motion is done in a smooth and controlled manner and that your feet remain parallel, with your knees bent directly over your toes. This will decrease sheering forces in the knees that can cause injury.

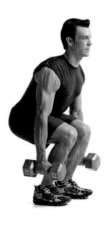

Wide-Feet Squats
Focus: **Thighs and buttocks**

Start: Stand tall with your feet more than shoulder-width apart and your toes angled outward about 45 degrees. Place your hands on your hips.

Action: Bend at your knees, placing your weight on your heels, and lower your thighs until they are no lower than parallel to the floor, ensuring your knees are bent directly over your toes. Return to the start position and repeat for the designated number of repetitions.

Trainer's Tip: Your toe and knee angle throughout this exercise is determined by your hip flexibility. Adjust your foot position based on your hip flexibility so that your knees are bent over your toes on every repetition.

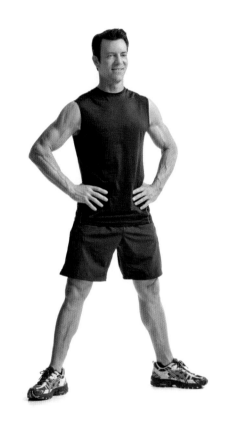

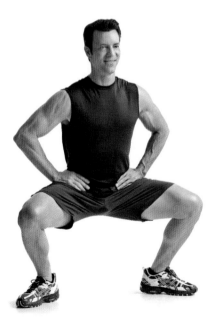

Speed Squats
Focus: **Thighs and buttocks**

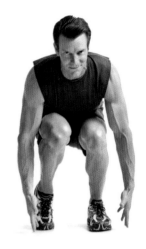

Start: Stand with your feet about shoulder width-apart with 80 percent of your weight on your left leg and 20 percent on the ball of the foot of your right leg. Assume a deep squat position with your chest and eyes up and fingertips touching the floor.

Action: In a quick and controlled movement, push off your left leg (your right foot is for balance only) to a standing position and extend both arms overhead. Quickly return to the start position and repeat for the designated number of repetitions.

Switch your foot position and repeat on your opposite leg.

Trainer's Tip: Speed and pace of this exercise are determined by your flexibility, range of motion, and athletic ability. Adjust the speed and depth of the squat based on your level of fitness.

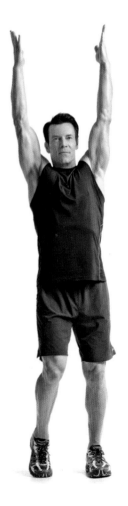

Wall Squats
Focus: **Thighs**

Start: Lean with your back against a strong and sturdy wall and lower yourself into a squat position. Your feet and knees should be shoulder-width apart, and your thighs should be parallel to the floor. Sit tall with your head against the wall and your ankles directly under your knees.

Action: Hold the start position for as long as you can.

Trainer's Tip: Clear your mind and breathe.

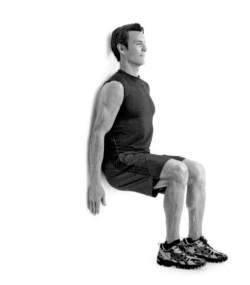

Screamer Lunges
Focus: **Thighs, buttocks, and abs**

Start: Step forward into a deep lunge with your left leg, keeping your right leg straightened behind you. Hold your arms out in front of you, elbows bent, with your hands clasped.

Action: Stay low and pull your right knee into your clasped hands, then return it to the start position as quickly as possible. Repeat for the designated number of repetitions, then switch legs and repeat.

Trainer's Tip: Stay low and move quickly for maximum effectiveness.

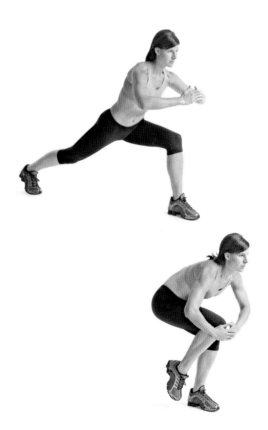

Pike Press with Leg Raises
Focus: Shoulders, triceps, buttocks, and hamstrings

Start: Place two dumbbells on the floor slightly more than shoulder-width apart. Get into a standard pushup position with your hands on the handles of the dumbbells. Walk your feet to your hands until your body is in the shape of a capital A. From this position, keep your legs straight, arms straight out, and core engaged.

Action: Keeping your right leg straight, raise it as high as you can behind you, then bend your arms and lower the crown of your head to about 1 inch from the ground between your hands. Straighten your arms while keeping your leg straight up behind you.

Switch legs and repeat on the opposite side to complete 1 rep, then continue for the designated number of repetitions.

Trainer's Tip: It's okay if you're unable to drop your head all the way to the floor. It's more important to find a range of motion that allows you to perform this exercise to the best of your ability.

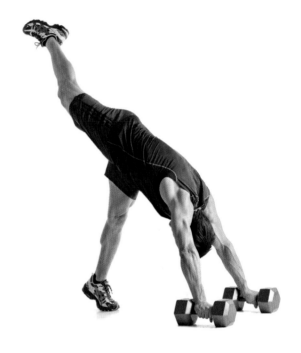

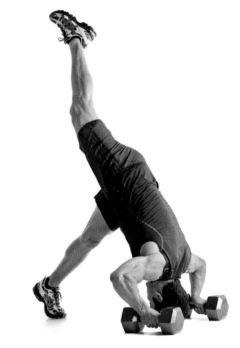

Tony's Motivators: Fitness Makes Life Easy

I'm learning that when you decide to eat right and exercise regularly, the person you become will have it pretty easy, and life will no longer seem quite as hard. Until I got really fit, I used to have so many problems. Everything seemed difficult and daunting. There was a lot of drama and conflict. I was lazy, tired, and overwhelmed. I didn't have the feel-good brain chemistry of a person who was firing on all cylinders from making better choices. Life was a struggle. But I had no clue that my poor diet and erratic physical activity were the reasons for my misery.

In my late twenties and early thirties, I began to eat better and work out more regularly. Oddly enough, new opportunities began to come my way. My confidence improved, and the drama began to fade away. It never occurred to me that healthier food and physical activity were responsible for the shifts in my life. I chalked it all up to luck, nothing more. Sometimes, for brief periods of time, I'd get lazy, eat garbage, and blow off workouts. And guess what? Life got hard again. But I still hadn't put two and two together.

By the time I made fitness my true vocation 13 years ago, I was in much better shape—not perfect, but pretty good. Those early days of creating my at-home DVD routines were fun and exciting. I was in the right place at the right time with the right experience to be able to help my business partners create something different and better when it came to at-home workouts. We were striking gold where it had never been found before. You'd think by then I'd have a clearer understanding that my regular exercise and healthy eating had something to do with my early triumphs, but the answer was still no. More great luck, right?

Turns out that the more consistent I was with my workouts and the better I ate, the more opportunities came my way. Only in the last 2 or 3 years have I truly begun to appreciate that by exercising 6 or 7 days a week and eating wholesome foods I have the energy and enthusiasm for a life I enjoy.

I'm not telling you this to brag—I'm sharing this experience because I want you to realize that life can be incredible, and not through luck or upbringing or even education. I know plenty of people who have degrees from top schools and who make tons of money—and they're a mess. Joy, happiness, opportunities, success, and the life you want come from switching to a lifestyle that involves regular exercise and whole foods. What seems hard as hell at first will turn your life into a carefree world of endless experiences and plenty of opportunities, and will give you the energy and enthusiasm needed to enjoy life for the rest of your life.

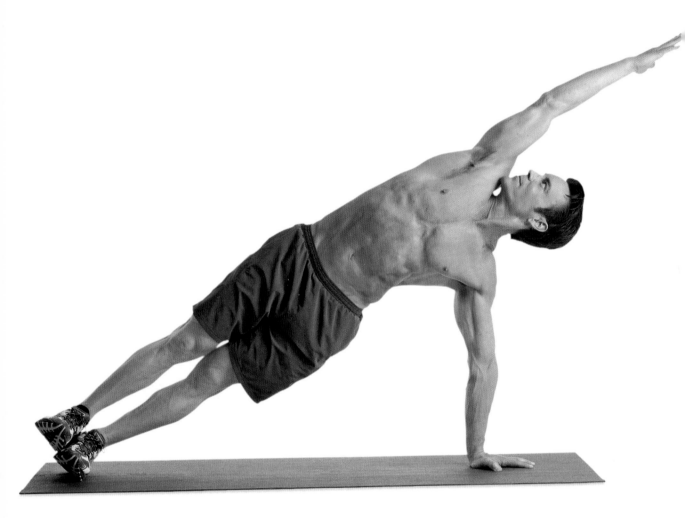

12

Hard Core

I don't know anyone, including me, who doesn't

want a six-pack, an eight-pack, or just plain flat abs. Sure, deeply chiseled abs look great and will get you lots of looks at the beach, but if you play sports or want a highly functional physique, a well-defined midsection is only half the story. The other half has to do with a strong core.

The term *core* (considered the epicenter of the body) applies to the muscle compartments of the abdominal area and lower back: the transverse abdominis (a deep corset of muscle that wraps around the torso and has much to do with breathing), rectus abdominis (your six-pack muscle), internal obliques (side muscles), and spinal erectors (lower back muscles). All work together, often simultaneously, to stabilize and support the spine.

Why is it important to build a strong core? There are several reasons. For one thing, it's the first step toward gaining strength and power and performing any kind of skilled athletic movement. You've probably heard the cliché "A chain is only as strong as its weakest link." For too many people, the weakest link in the body is this crucial center of power, agility, and balance. When your core is strong, your whole body benefits. My program places a high priority on developing core strength, since neglecting these important muscles can create a weak link at the body's center.

Second, a strong core, especially the supporting muscles around the spine, can help minimize and prevent lower back pain, as well as reduce the risk of lower back injury. Science has already weighed in on the importance of this: A review study conducted by the Yoga Research Foundation looked into the value of yoga as a treatment for lower back pain. Yoga is one of my favorite forms of exercise, and it focuses greatly on core strength. Eighty people did either yoga or calisthenics-type exercises (this was the control group) for just 1 week, and the results were rather amazing: Just 7 days of yoga reduced back pain and improved spinal flexibility better than the other exercise program.[1]

Finally, because the core encompasses all the abdominal muscles that make up that sexy six-pack look, a strong core is the foundation for a ripped midsection (though you may need to clean up your diet to see it). This benefit is more than cosmetic: At a time when abdominal fat has been linked to problems with obesity, cardiovascular disease, diabetes, and kidney ailments, doctors are encouraging men and women to tackle abdominal weight gain before it grows into a major problem. And, according to a recent study in the journal *Neurology*, people with smaller waistlines are up to three times less likely to develop dementia as those with larger ones. Carrying extra belly fat, even if you're at a healthy weight, may boost the production of hormones that damage blood vessels in the brain and heart.[2]

I am often asked, "What's the best ab exercise?" It's tough for me to label any one exercise as being the "best" for building a particular muscle group, especially since variety is a critical component of muscle development. For that reason, I'll offer you a variety of core exercises. They all improve posture and enhance movements used for daily activities and athletic performance. They also strengthen and define abdominal and lower back muscles, which help to flatten the tummy and decrease excess back fat.

BOSU Fun

One of my favorite pieces of equipment is the BOSU (rhymes with "tofu," sort of) ball. It took me a little while to be won over by it, but when I heard it was useful for skiers (and others) who need to work on balance, I got interested. Balance is essential for snow-sport skills.

A BOSU ball looks like a stability ball that has been cut in half. It has an inflated dome on one side and is flat on the other. It's low-tech, but it challenges different body systems appropriately to improve balance and stability. I learned that it could be used for a lot of core exercises, such as crunches. It's so much fun and a great piece of exercise equipment. It makes me feel like a kid again. Once I started using it, I could see a dozen ways to use it in my personal training gym. My clients have never forgiven me.

If you stand on top of the dome, thus creating a compromise to your balance, it really challenges your muscles. If you flip it over, you can use it to do pushups. You can also stand on the BOSU ball while simultaneously lifting dumbbells—a protocol referred to as "unstable surface training." A 2007 study in the *Journal of Strength and Conditioning Research* looked at the chest press specifically and found that key muscles in the back and abdomen might work anywhere from two to seven times as hard when the upper body, lower body, or both are rendered unstable.[3]

However you use it, the BOSU helps fire up all the major muscle groups, plus smaller muscles, and improves your balance. And it's fun!

Besides the specific core moves described in this chapter, other exercises in my program strengthen the core as well. Basic pushups and pullups strengthen your core, because unlike workouts done on elaborate machinery in gyms, body weight–bearing exercises like these involve stability and balance—which are jobs for your core muscles.

The other question I get asked a lot has to do with all the ab-training gizmos on the market and whether they work. I love the tried-and-true—crunches, bicycles, twists, and so forth. That's what works for me and my clients. Several years ago, I was glad to see that a study conducted by scientists from California State University, Northridge, backed me up on this. The study offered proof that abdominal exercisers claiming to aerobically burn fat and flatten your stomach "in just minutes a day" are no more effective than traditional, unaided crunch exercises.

The researchers arrived at their conclusion by monitoring 25 men and women between the ages of 18 and 40 as they performed various exercises with an ab gizmo and then compared the results with their performance using more traditional exercises like the crunch, oblique crunch, and trunk extension. The results, published in the *Journal of Physical Education, Recreation, and Dance*, indicated that overall, the gizmo generated less muscle activity than the traditional moves. The researchers also found that use of the gizmo produced an average heart rate that wasn't high enough to trigger much fat burning. All research results confirmed that working out with this piece of trendy equipment didn't produce quick results, despite the manufacturer's claims, and that traditional abdominal exercises are still the most effective (at least in terms of generating muscle activity).[4]

When you use a variety of my core moves (which require no equipment except maybe an optional BOSU ball), expect to see a big difference in the tone and definition of your body in about 6 weeks and in your posture in about 3 weeks. You'll also build a strong and supportive lower back. By training your core muscles, you'll improve strength, stability, and power. An added bonus: Your body will appear leaner and tighter as you work those deeper midsection muscles.

Crunches
Focus: **Upper abdominals**

Start: Lie on your back. Bend your knees and place your feet flat on the floor about hip-width apart. Place your hands behind your head just behind your ears (do not clasp your hands together).

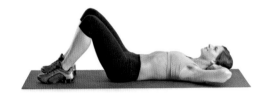

Action: Lift your shoulders off the floor, keeping your chin off your chest and your elbows wide (do not pull on your head with your hands). Repeat for the designated number of repetitions.

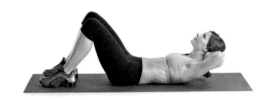

Trainer's Tip: Be sure to press your lower back into the floor at the top of the crunch—this creates a neutral spine, which is important to maintain throughout the exercise.

In and Out Crunches
Focus: **Upper and lower abdominals**

Start: Lie on your back with your feet together, legs extended, and hands behind your head (do not clasp your hands together) with your elbows wide.

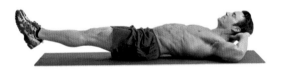

Action: Lift your shoulder blades and feet off the floor, then bend your knees in toward your chest and lift your upper body in a standard crunch. Return to the previous position (with your shoulder blades and feet off the floor) and repeat for the designated number of repetitions.

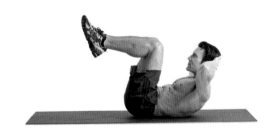

Trainer's Tip: Beginners can modify this movement by resting their heels and shoulders on the floor between repetitions.

Scissor Crunches
Focus: **Upper and lower abdominals**

Start: Lie on your back with your feet together, legs extended, and hands behind your head (do not clasp your hands together) with your elbows wide. Raise your right foot straight up to the ceiling and keep your left leg extended and your left foot a few inches from the floor.

Action: From the start position, perform a standard crunch, then lower your upper body to about an inch from the floor and switch legs. Repeat the crunch and continue the sequence for the designated number of repetitions.

Trainer's Tip: Beginners can modify this movement by gently resting one foot and their upper body on the floor between repetitions.

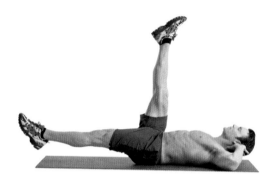

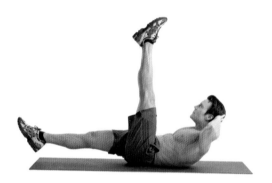

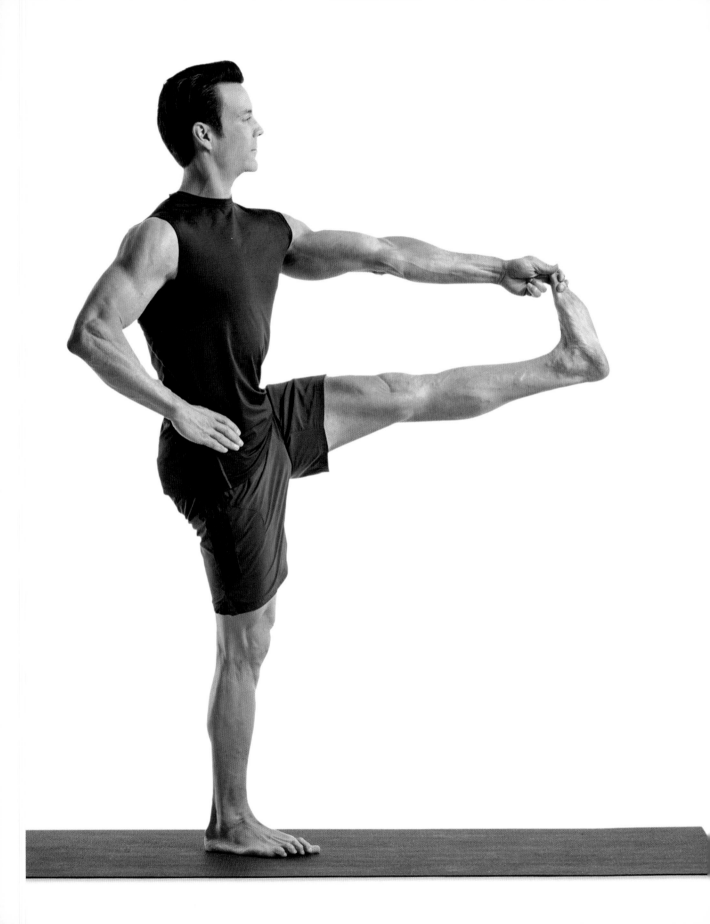

13

Flex Appeal

Want to feel and look young again? Outlive the

Harry Potter or James Bond sequels? Researchers are discovering that just about every aspect of aging is affected by our lifestyles. While genetics still plays a big part, it's very much up to you whether you'll keel over before you receive your AARP card in the mail or hang around long enough to spoil your great-grandkids. And one of the best ways to live to an old-yet-active age is to stay flexible through stretching and an active lifestyle.

Every year after the age of 35, we lose 1 percent of our flexibility. Therefore, by age 65, we will be 30 percent less limber. As we age, the elasticity of tendons, ligaments, and joint capsules decreases as collagen fibers in those tissues cross-link, or "mat," together. Our bodies then feel like brittle old bleach bottles.

Eventually, this process shortens the belly of each of your muscles, causing them to tire out a lot faster. A loss of flexibility with age may also be the result of certain diseases, such as arthritis.

Poor flexibility inhibits each muscle from working through the most complete range of motion possible, which denies you the maximum benefits of your workouts. But if you regularly stretch, you can increase your range of motion, and as a result, your muscles may produce even greater force. This is because a stretched muscle has the potential to exert more force than a tight muscle. And when you don't stretch properly, inflexible tendons and other connective tissues can shrink. This increases the likelihood of pulling them, leading to pain and injury and leaving you sidelined from exercise or any other activity. And when you're not active, your muscles and ligaments become even weaker and thus more prone to injury from everyday activity. It's a vicious cycle.

Staying limber and flexible through stretching and exercise is the way to prevent all of this from happening, which is why I always say: Flexibility is the fountain of youth!

Back in the 1960s (yes, I'm that old), we took fitness tests in school that were meant to determine how fit we were: pushups, pullups, dips, situps (not crunches), the 100-yard dash, and touching your toes. The first five items were used to measure strength and speed. Some kids had it, while others did not. I was in the "did not" category. (That changed later.) Touching your toes was a breeze for all of us. Even out-of-shape kids like me could touch their toes.

When you're young (no matter what kind of shape you're in), you're naturally flexible and durable. Kids get scrapes, bruises, even broken bones, but it's pretty rare for young children to pull a muscle, and if they do, they recover in the blink of an eye. Back in the good old days, the focus was on running faster and jumping higher. The only kids in my neighborhood who stretched were gymnasts or ballerinas. Try to imagine a stretch class for children in the 1960s. Yeah, right!

In those days, proper stretching didn't happen. For most adults, it still doesn't. You may not like it because you think it's boring; maybe it even makes you grimace. Stretching cuts into your workout time, but deep down you know it's good for you. It will make you more pliable, plus make your muscles function better, behave "younger," and become more injury resistant. Stretching also helps you get better results from resistance training. All that, *and* it takes only a few minutes, requires no equipment, has no harmful side effects, and doesn't cost a penny.

I'm here to tell you that it's time to rethink the importance of flexibility.

Stretch for Success

Each one of my workouts incorporates stretching as part of the warmup and the cooldown. I've even slipped a few yoga moves into the routines.

It's important to warm up and stretch before beginning your intense workout. When you elevate your body and muscle temperatures by warming up, a lot of temperature-related changes occur inside your body. Blood flow to and from your muscles increases, which means more energy sources (like blood sugar) are delivered and more metabolic by-products (lactic acid) are removed. Hemoglobin and myoglobin (extra sources of oxygen in skeletal muscle) relay more energy-giving oxygen to your muscles. The friction inside your muscle fibers is reduced, which improves their mechanical efficiency. The transmission speed of nerve impulses, which cause your muscle fibers to contract, increases. Your metabolic rate is elevated, which means you burn more calories. A good warmup is the foundation of a great workout.

You'll conclude your workout with a cooldown—at least 5 to 10 minutes of light cardio and stretches to gradually return your body to its warmup state and heart rate.

Here are some guidelines to help you stretch for success.

Always warm up. Before stretching anything, warm up with some light cardio for about 5 minutes to elevate your body temperature. At the start of a workout, your body is like cold taffy. If you try to bend it, it breaks. But let it warm up, and it becomes a soft cloth you can fold. It's the same with your muscles. When they're cold, they're stiff and inflexible, and forcibly stretching them could lead to injury or strains. But warm them up and you can touch your toes and maybe even kiss your kneecaps.

Take your time. Hold each stretch for a minimum of 10 seconds and progressively work your way up to 20 seconds or more.

Take deep breaths while you stretch. Breathing deeply helps you to relax, furthering your stretch and therefore your flexibility.

Don't let it hurt. Stretching shouldn't be painful. In the beginning, you will notice some minor discomfort as you stretch inflexible muscles. If you feel pain, you're likely pushing yourself too far.

Be patient. It took you years to achieve your stiff, brittle condition, so don't expect to be Gumby overnight. Be diligent and consistent with your flexibility goals and you'll see results fairly quickly.

Make it a habit. The main reason people don't become more flexible is because they're not willing to put in the time. The axiom for other aspects of fitness also applies to flexibility: You get better at the things you do often. Stretching and yoga are equally as important as strength conditioning and cardiovascular fitness. Integrate flexibility work into your daily fitness program. It takes only 10 to 15 minutes a day and can be done before or after your exercise routine. And hey, you could even make a few bucks the next time someone bets that you can't touch your toes to the back of your head.

Yoga for Optimum Flexibility

Hearing the word *yoga* as a kid, I thought people were mispronouncing "yogurt." Come to think of it, I didn't know what yogurt was, either. Some kind of healthy sour milk? Ew. (I love it now!)

Developed in ancient India as far back as 5,000 years ago, yoga employs bodily postures (asanas), breathing techniques (pranayama), and meditation (dhyana) with the goal of bringing about a sound, healthy body and a clear, calm mind. What began as a spiritual pursuit has become a more corporeal matter in its American incarnation. Today's yoga enthusiasts tend to seek proper posture, heart health, stress reduction, and even weight loss, although the spiritual benefits still permeate the discipline and generate interest. In practicing the hundreds of physical poses, you will not only gain strength and flexibility but also join your mind and body in a way that benefits overall well-being.

As you do yoga, you'll find that, like anything else, you get out of it what you put into it. You'd never go to a music lesson once a week without practicing and expect to play well. The same goes for yoga. Try establishing a home practice of as little as 10 minutes a day. Sample my yoga routines; they assist you in progressing from Beginner's yoga to Striver's yoga to Warrior's yoga.

Over the years, I've discovered that yoga makes everything else I do easier, from sports to all other workouts. Yoga also brings a mental aspect to physical movement that heightens my awareness and appreciation for my overall health and fitness. If you choose to practice yoga, I promise, you'll feel energized, invigorated, and maybe even a little enlightened. Who wouldn't want all of those benefits?

Stretching and yoga can help restore the natural flexibility and durability of our younger years. Flexibility is the fountain of youth. Give yourself that amazing gift. Here's to touching your toes.

My Basic Stretches

Side Stretch

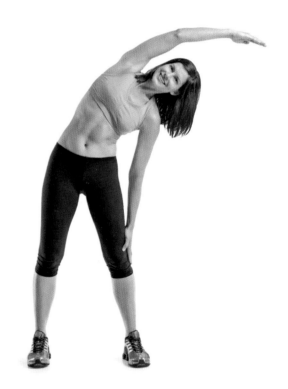

Start: Stand with your feet slightly more than shoulder-width apart.

Action: From the start position, inhale, then exhale, as you bend to the left, reaching your right hand over your head, stretching the right side of your body. As your reach overhead with your right hand, slide your left hand down your left leg.

Hold this position for 3 full breaths. After your third breath, exhale both arms up over your head as you return to an upright position. Inhale with your arms at the top and exhale as you repeat the movement to your right, stretching your left side.

Repeat 3 times on each side.

Trainer's Tip: Never hold your breath during this movement. Rest your hand lightly on your leg and be careful not to press on your knee.

Arm Circles

Start: Stand with your feet shoulder-width apart, one foot slightly behind the other. Raise your arms out to your sides (parallel to the floor), fingertips pointed toward the ceiling.

Action: While maintaining the start position, rotate your arms clockwise in 6-inch-circles for 20 repetitions, then repeat in a counter-clockwise direction.

Trainer's Tip: Breathe! Never hold your breath during stretches.

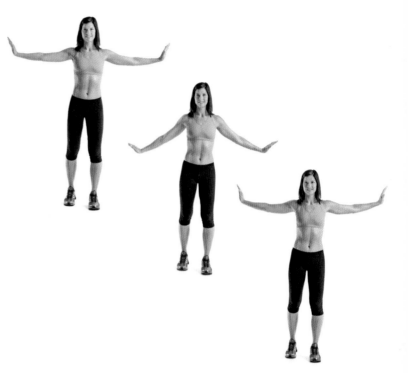

Standing Quad Stretch

Start: Stand on one foot, keeping the knee of the leg you're standing on slightly bent.

Action: Bend the other knee and, using the same-side hand, grab the top of your foot and pull it up toward your buttocks. Stand tall, keep your knees close together, and push your hips slightly forward.

Hold this position for 3 full, slow breaths, then switch legs and repeat.

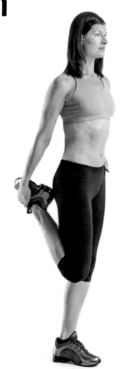

Split-Leg Hamstring Stretch

Start: Stand with your feet together, then step back with your right foot so that it's about 2 feet behind your left foot. Your heels should be aligned front to back, with the toes of your left foot forward and the toes of your right foot pointed slightly outward, and your upper inner thighs should be touching.

Action: Flex the muscles in your thighs, forcing both legs to be perfectly straight, and then begin to collapse your upper body down over your front leg. While in this position, turn your right hip forward and left hip back.

Hold this position for 5 full, deep breaths. Carefully bend your front leg, engage your core, and return to the start position. Repeat on the opposite side.

Trainer's Tip: Do not bend your knees. Lower your upper body as far as you can, but don't force this stretch just to get your hands on the floor.

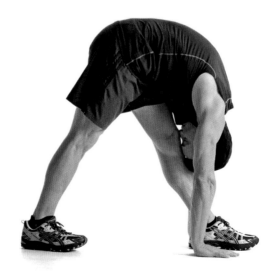

Runner's Stretch

Start: Get into a lunge position with your left knee bent and right leg as straight as possible. Make sure that your front knee is directly over your ankle (of the front foot).

Action: Place your hands on the floor on the inside of your left foot, then drop your pelvis as low as you can while keeping your back leg as straight as you can.

Hold this position for 5 full, deep breaths and then change legs.

Advanced Runner's Stretch: Lower your torso and place your forearms on the floor, still keeping your back leg as straight as possible. Perform the exercise as instructed above. Note: As part of the Warrior's Yoga Routine on page 82, this movement is referred to as Advanced Runner's Pose.

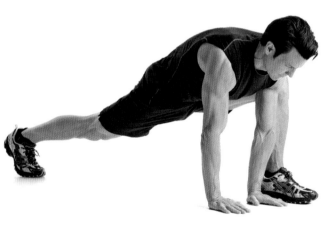

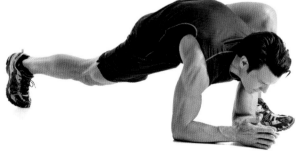

Head Rolls

Start: Stand with your feet about shoulder-width apart and your arms at your sides.

Action: Gently lower your chin forward and hold it there for 10 seconds.

Then slowly roll your head to the left, backward, and to the right. Hold for 10 seconds, then switch directions. Alternate 4 times to each side.

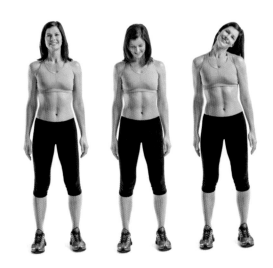

Shoulder Rolls

Start: Stand with your feet about shoulder-width apart.

Action: Shrug your shoulders up and slowly roll them forward and down, then back and up—as if you are moving them in a circle.

Repeat the sequence for 8 repetitions. Reverse the direction of the shoulder rolls and repeat.

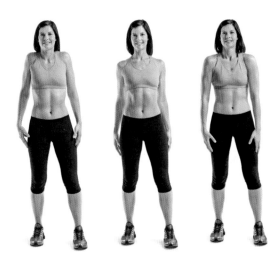

Double Backstroke

Start: Stand with your feet about shoulder-width apart, one leg slightly forward. Extend your arms out to your sides.

Action: Simulate the backstroke by: moving your arms back and down, to the front, up, down, and back in one single fluid movement.

Return to the start position. Repeat for the designated number of repetitions.

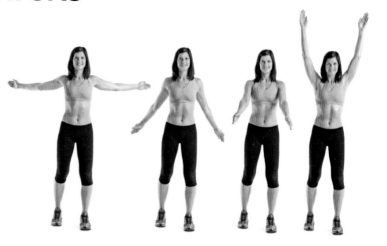

Double Front Stroke

Start: Stand with your feet about shoulder-width apart, one leg slightly forward. Extend your arms out to your sides.

Action: Bring your arms up above your head, down in front of your body, back, and back up to your sides in one single fluid movement.

Repeat for the designated number of repetitions.

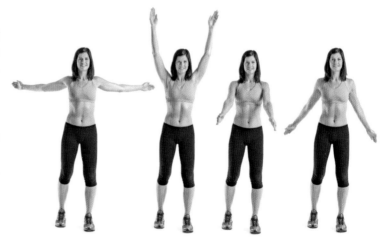

Huggers

Start: Stand with your feet close together, one foot slightly behind the other, and your arms extended out to your sides and parallel to the floor.

Action: Quickly throw your arms around your torso in a hugging motion, then quickly open and release your arms as wide as possible. Throw your arms around your torso again, switching top-arm position, then open and release to complete 1 rep.

Repeat the complete sequence for 20 repetitions.

Trainer's Tip: This ballistic stretch is different than traditional static stretches. It is designed to warm up ligaments, tendons, and connective tissue more than muscle.

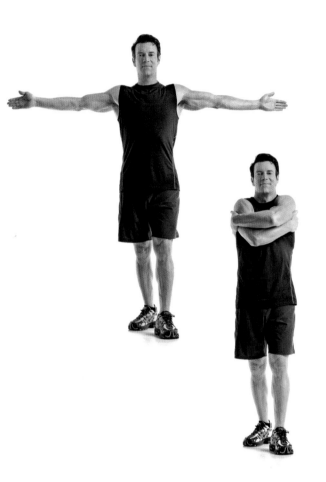

Chest Stretch

Start: Stand with your feet close together, one foot slightly behind the other. Reach your arms up overhead with your fingers spread apart.

Action: Keeping your fingers spread, begin to bend your elbows and lower them to just below chest level. Be sure to pull your elbows back as you descend. Return to the start position and repeat for 5 repetitions.

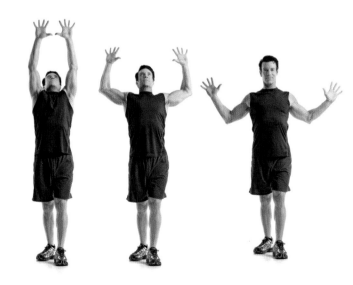

My Yoga Moves

Yoga Hamstring Stretch

Start: Stand straight and tall with your feet hip-width apart, arms at your sides, and feet parallel.

Action: Inhale your arms straight overhead, arch your back slightly, then exhale, folding forward at the hips. Keep your legs straight, relax your head, and hang down. Hold the bottom position for 5 deep breaths.

Variations: You can do the pose to your left leg, right leg, and with your feet wide apart for a different stretch on your spine and legs.

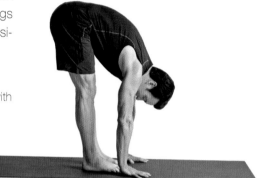

Seated Twist

Start: Sit on your left hip and thigh, with your left knee pointing forward and your left foot beneath your right buttocks. Place your right foot flat on the floor next to your left thigh.

Action: Place your left elbow just below your right knee and your right hand on the floor slightly behind you. Inhale deeply and, as you exhale, gently twist to look behind you, pressing your left elbow against your right thigh.

Deepen the twist by continuing to take 4 deep breaths and pressing your elbow against your thigh, then switch legs and repeat on the opposite side.

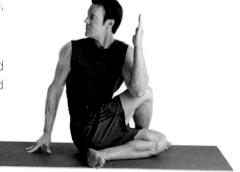

Child's Pose

Start: Kneel on the floor with your knees slightly wider than hip-width apart and your big toes touching behind you.

Action: Fold forward bringing your forehead down onto the floor. Reach forward with both arms, placing palms flat on the floor for an added shoulder stretch.

Relax your body forward and be sure to inhale and exhale deeply for 5 full breaths.

Trainer's Tip: Stay in this pose for as long as you like.

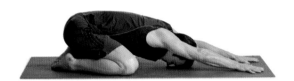

Mountain Pose

Start: Stand tall with your feet together and arms down with your palms forward.

Action: Gently squeeze your buttocks, tilt your pelvis forward, relax your shoulders, spread your toes, and keep your weight in your heels as you reach the crown of your head toward the ceiling. Close your eyes and breathe deeply in and out.

Hold this position for 5 deep breaths.

Note: Refer to the second photo for an alternative hand position.

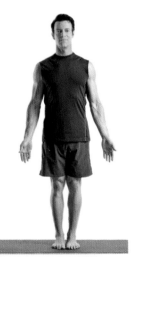
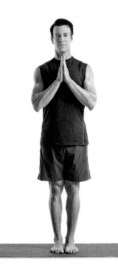

Forward Bend

Start: Stand tall in Mountain Pose with feet hip-width apart.

Action: Inhale and bring both arms up tall overhead. Exhale while bending at the waist, keeping your legs straight and core engaged, and collapse forward into a forward bend. Relax your head (especially your neck) and entire torso while hanging forward as low as you can. Remain here for 1 or 2 breaths.

Advanced Forward Bend Hamstring Stretch: Form Forward Bend, with your feet hip-width apart, reach both hands behind the base of both calves. Bring your forearms and elbows close to your legs as you reach your fingertips to the floor. Pull your torso and face lower and closer to your legs. Hold for 5 breaths.

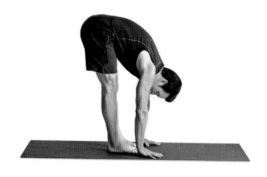

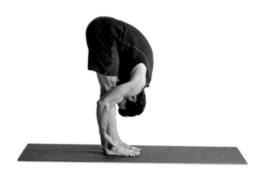

Flat Back (Partial Sun Salute)

Start: From Forward Bend.

Action: Keeping your legs straight, inhale and bring your torso, head, and arms away from the floor up to a flat-back position. Exhale and return to the bottom position of Forward Bend.

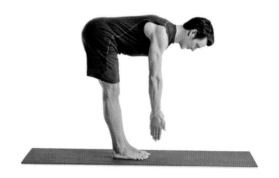

Plank Pose

Start: From Forward Bend.

Action: Step or gently float your feet back to the start position of a pushup (also known as Plank Pose). Keep your arms straight with your hands shoulder-width apart, fingers spread. Squeeze your buttocks, tilt your pelvis forward, and engage your abdominals. Look forward slightly.

Hold this position for a breath or two.

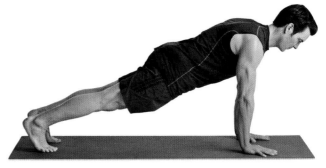

Chataranga

Start: From Plank Pose.

Action: Keeping your body strong and rigid, lower yourself to the bottom of a military-style pushup (elbows close to your sides). Your chest should be a few inches from the floor, and your eyes should remain looking forward.

Hold for 1 breath.

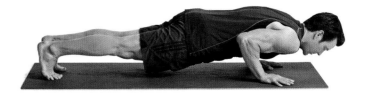

Upward-Facing Dog

Start: From bottom position of Chataranga.

Action: Keeping your hands shoulder-width apart, arms straight and perpendicular to the floor, and wrists directly beneath your shoulders, lift the crown of your head as high as possible, roll onto the top of your feet, relax your back and pelvis, and look straight ahead.

Hold for 1 or 2 breaths.

Note: If keeping your knees off the floor is too difficult, bend your elbows and rest your knees on the floor. This is called Cobra Pose.

Trainer's Tip: Upward-Facing Dog is a preparatory move leading to Plank Pose, then Downward-Facing Dog.

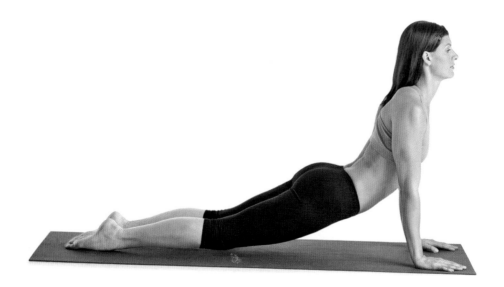

Downward-Facing Dog

Start: From Plank Pose.

Action: Raise your buttocks straight into the air; your heels will begin to move closer to the floor. Try to keep your hands and feet from moving closer together as you transition from Plank Pose to Downward-Facing Dog.

Turn your heels out slightly and continue to spread your fingers, driving your chest down toward the floor and fighting to keep your arms straight as you continue to drive your buttocks skyward. Do your best to align your ears with your biceps.

Hold this position for 3 or 4 breaths.

Trainer's Tip: For an additional calf and Achilles stretch, pedal your feet during the breathing sequence, lifting one heel and pushing down with the other. Hold each position for a full breath, then switch.

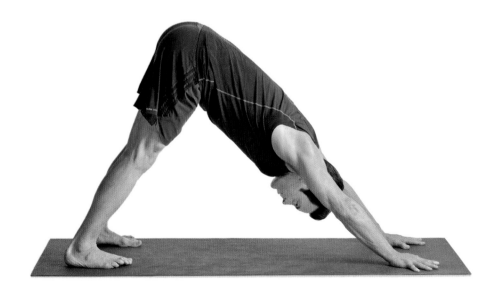

Runner's Pose

Start: From Downward-Facing Dog.

Action: Lower your buttocks and step your left foot forward into a lunge so that your left anklebone is directly beneath your left knee. Your right leg should be straight and sturdy as you drive the back heel toward the floor.

Lift your chest away from your thigh and move your hands so that your fingertips are just grazing the floor. Your arms are straight and perpendicular to the floor. Look forward slightly so that your spine is aligned from your head through your torso.

Hold this position for 3 breaths, then repeat on the opposite side.

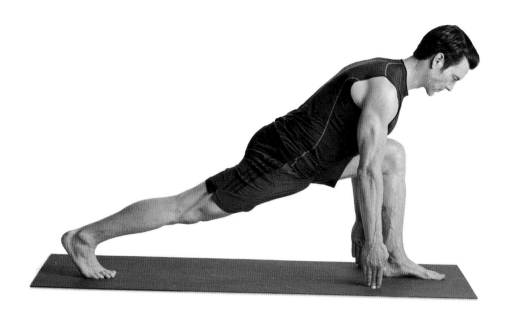

Crescent Pose

Start: From Runner's Pose.

Action: Using the strength of both legs while engaging your core muscles, slowly lift your fingers away from the floor in a forward-sweeping motion until your torso is tall and your arms are reaching skyward. Try to maintain a deep lunge so your front thigh is parallel to the floor, knee remains over your ankle, arms are straight (next to your ears), and shoulders are relaxed with your back leg straight and strong.

Hold this position for 3 breaths, then repeat on the opposite side.

Trainer's Tip: Keeping your back leg straight is key, so focus on lifting the back of your knee toward the ceiling and simultaneously driving your heel toward the floor while remaining on the ball of your back foot.

Standing Leg Extension

Start: Stand tall with your feet hip-width apart and hands on your hips.

Action: Place 90 percent of your weight on your right foot with your right leg straight or slightly bent. Transition all your weight to your right leg as you begin to lift your left leg off the floor.

Extend your left leg straight out in front of you (attempting to make your thigh parallel to the floor), flex your left foot, and grab your big toe with your middle and index fingers of your left hand. Keep your right hand on your right hip.

Hold this position for 5 breaths, then repeat on the opposite side.

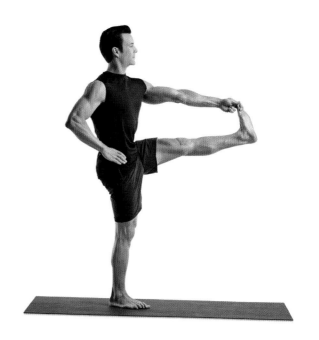

Pigeon Pose

Start: Get on your hands and knees.

Action: Pull your right knee to the outside of your right wrist with your foot flexed and your shin and ankle making contact with the floor. Extend your left leg straight behind you so that the top of your foot and knee make contact with the floor. Stay here, or begin to bring your torso and forehead down toward the floor with your arms and torso reaching out in front of you.

Hold this position for 10 full breaths, then repeat on the opposite side.

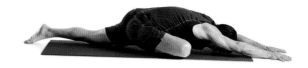

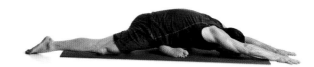

Crane Pose

Start: From a crouched position, place your hands shoulder-width apart on the floor. Open your knees wider than your elbows and press the inside of your knees against upper arms.

Action: Shift your weight onto your hands and slowly lift one foot at a time off the floor until you find your balance point.

Hold this position for 5 breaths or as long as you can maintain your balance.

Note: This movement can be performed either with arms bent or straight. The straight arm version is more difficult.

Trainer's Tip: Engaging your core muscles will help you learn this balance pose more quickly.

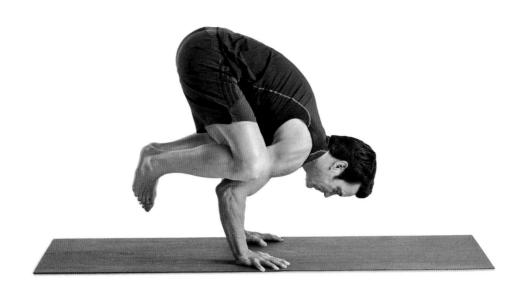

Reverse Warrior

Start: From Warrior II.

Action: While remaining low in your lunge, reach back and place your right hand on your straight, strong right leg. Simultaneously lean back and reach your left arm over your head toward the wall behind you. Turn your chin into your raised arm and look past your hand.

Hold for 3 breaths, then repeat on the opposite side.

Trainer's Tip: Avoid placing too much weight on the back leg with your hand. Try to rest your hand lightly on the leg to avoid placing too much pressure on your knee, and be sure to keep your front knee bent in a deep lunge.

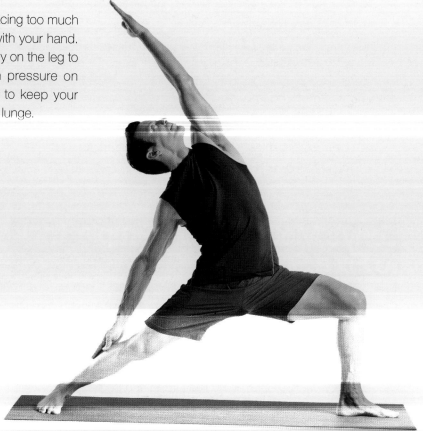

Corpse Pose (Savasana)

Start: Lie on your back on the floor with your feet hip-width apart and relaxed, arms comfortably by your sides, and palms up. A time for breathing and reflection.

Action: None. Just breathe.

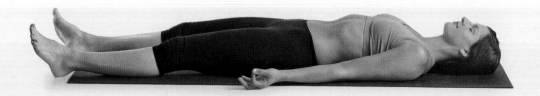

Tony's Motivators: A Simple Trick to Fix a Stiff Back

If you experience unexplained stiffness and tightness in your lower back on a regular basis, try adopting this simple habit that will improve your lower back and core strength: When you walk, focus on your ab and glute muscles and keep them strong. You don't have to put a lot of energy into this. Just constantly flex your behind and abdominal areas while you go about your business. The key is to consciously use your gluteal and abdominal muscles whenever you stand, walk, jog, and run. If you do this correctly, your gait will feel strong and purposeful, you will become more aware of the muscles that surround your hip and lower back areas, and your lower back pain will diminish.

PART 4 The Meal Plan

I've always been a wannabe jock. When I was a kid, football, Frisbee, tennis, basketball, skiing, and hockey (on ponds and lakes) were my favorite sports. I thought I ate okay, but then again I thought a fluffernutter (peanut butter and marshmallow creme on white bread) was a decent meal. The truth is, I didn't have a clue about balancing exercise and proper diet. I ran around like most kids in the 1960s and 1970s, burning calories but eating a diet loaded with fat, sugar, and salt.

A brief meal plan from the young-man Horton days:

Breakfast: A bowl of Cocoa Krispies, Cap'n Crunch, or Lucky Charms, swimming in whole milk, followed by a double order of cinnamon toast with butter.

Lunch: A sandwich heaped with a variety of processed meats on white bread (always) with tons of mayo; an ice cream sandwich or two with a Twinkie made the ideal double dessert. No wonder I fell asleep in fifth-period math!

Dinner: Spaghetti and meatballs, pork or lamb chops, pizza, steak and potatoes, meat loaf, lasagna, barbecued chicken and corn on the cob, and so on. My mom was a great cook, and these were the recipes she prepared for our family for years. I don't recall eating much fruit or many fresh vegetables because I'd eat only the salty canned and frozen varieties.

Who knew, right? Certainly not me at that young age, and forget about any nutrition classes in those days. It took a shattered kneecap during my sophomore year in college—a casualty of skiing on a steep slope with too little snow and too many frozen tree stumps at Smugglers' Notch in northern Vermont—to help me realize the importance of a healthier diet. Through a rigorous physical therapy program, I began to discover the benefits—mental and physical—of healthy nutrition. Since that fateful injury, my diet slowly evolved into a health-changing regimen of lean protein, fruits and veggies, and complex carbohydrates.

People always ask me what I eat to maintain my fitness level and stay in peak health. First off, let me tell you what I *don't* eat: I steer clear of red meat or any processed (deli) meats and most dairy products. I stay away from "beige foods": Tater Tots, french fries, fried chicken, mashed potatoes, fish and chips, corn chips, and, of course, any and all processed foods. This fake food is nothing more than fatty, greasy, salty empty calories. Nasty stuff, if you ask me.

I eat fresh, whole, organic foods that compose the colors of the rainbow: green, purple, yellow, orange, and red. I eat lean proteins (wild-caught fish, free-range chicken) and tons of legumes (navy beans, kidney beans, chickpeas). You name a bean and I eat it. Protein, fiber, nutrients—it's all in there. Sweet potatoes are a staple. I find a way to put them in everything. My sandwiches include as many veggies as possible—tomatoes, cucumbers, lettuce, spinach, avocados, and peppers. When I eat bread, I choose high-fiber, whole-grain, or sprouted bread. And unlike high school Tony, I pass on the mayo: just mustard, please. This diet allows me to work out 6 or 7 days a week, sleep the appropriate 7½ to 8 hours a night, and have through-the-roof energy and vitality. This is how I advise my celebrity clients to eat, and it's how I want you to eat, too.

I trained Billy Idol—the notorious lip-curling bad-boy rocker known for his punk rock classics—in the late 1980s through the early 1990s. In February 1990, he had a near-fatal motorcycle accident that required five operations and threatened to end his career. He fractured his left forearm and suffered multiple fractures of and muscle damage to his lower right leg. While hospitalized, Billy was at the mercy of hospital nutritionists who wanted to fill him with red meat, processed carbs, high-fat proteins, and sugary desserts. That is, until I stepped in to quash that ridiculous approach with complex carbs, lean proteins, fruits, veggies, and a steady rehab program right there in his hospital bed. It worked for me after my knee injury, and I knew it would work for Billy. The results were rapid and amazing. He got back in top shape—and back on tour.

Overview: My Meal Plan

My Meal Plan is not a starvation diet—and it's probably a lot different from the plans you've tried before. Developed by my personal chef, Melissa Costello, it's a blend of brand-new and old-school. While it is designed to revitalize, replenish, and reenergize you, it is, in fact, probably not that different from how your great-grandparents ate 100 years ago. My Meal Plan is a commonsense, simple, nutrition-focused approach to improved health and weight loss. I tell my clients that if weight control is their sole focus, they're missing the point of eating healthy whole foods.

This plan is based on the "flexitarian" approach to diet. In general, that means eating a primarily plant-based diet focused on whole foods. This gives your body all of the nutritional building blocks it needs: high-fiber complex carbs; lean, healthy protein; tons of fruits and vegetables; and healthy fats for recovery, strength, energy, and optimal health and wellness.

There are three parts to my Meal Plan; they work hand in hand.

Part I: Cleanse. First, you'll gradually cleanse your system of toxins over a 30-day period, and in doing so, you'll encourage your body to function on a higher level. The cleanse isn't a fast; it's a system of phasing toxins from your system. I'll walk you through it in Chapter 14.

Part 2: Nourish. While you're cleansing, you'll eat from a prescribed list of highly nutritious foods: leafy greens and other vegetables, legumes, fruits, whole grains and pseudo-grains, nuts and seeds, dairy foods and dairy substitutes, lean organically produced proteins, and healthy fats. You'll learn more about this in Chapter 15.

Part 3: Supplement. My stand on supplements is that they work well, but only after your diet is squared away. After all, a supplement does just that: It supplements your diet. For some time, now, nutritional science has acknowledged that vitamins and minerals are not the only beneficial nutrients. In addition to vitamins and minerals, there are many other micronutrients that help your body function at its best and improve your performance and overall fitness. I'll outline those supplements in Chapter 16.

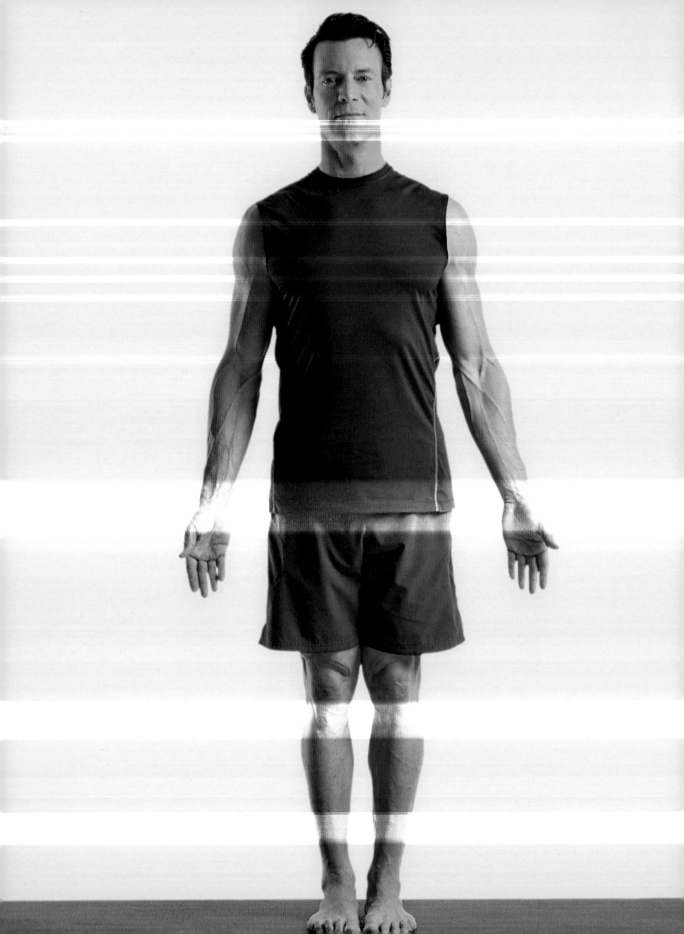

14

Part I: Cleanse

The "cleansing" part of my plan is accomplished

by the gradual elimination over a 30-day period of five substances: caffeine, alcohol, sugar and processed foods, gluten, and animal products. Does that list scare you? If so, it may mean you have an addiction to one or more of these "toxins." An addiction is something you're emotionally chained to. Your life is controlled by an outside substance, and you feel uncomfortable without it. If you think you can't live without caffeine, alcohol, or sugar, then this is the perfect time to get started and discover that you have complete control over your health and what you put in your body.

Now don't panic or be skeptical, either. The motivation to continue this plan will come from your own body. Why? Because you'll begin to feel a natural high a few days into the cleanse. You'll experience much-improved digestion and loads of energy. And any extra weight will start melting off naturally.

You'll implement all three components of the plan over 30 days. The sequence has been carefully planned to alter your body chemistry gradually and make it easier for you to stick to the new eating habits you're forming. After the 30-day period, you can add foods back in, if you want to, although the vast majority of people opt to stay with 100 percent "clean" eating or find that their taste buds have changed and they no longer desire caffeine, meat, sugar, or alcohol. The same foods that they craved and couldn't live without 30 days ago suddenly seem bland, too sweet, or just plain gross!

Here's a closer look at what you'll be phasing out and how to do it.

Alcohol

Over the course of the last 10 years, I've cut my alcohol consumption by 98 percent. I've never been a big drinker anyway, and even in college I limited my beer intake to weekends only. They were crazy college weekends, sure, that also included vomiting and hangovers. Ridiculous, when I think about it now. I used to drink for the same reasons most people do. I enjoyed the buzz, it helped me relax, it gave me courage when I needed it, and it allowed me to escape from the "real world" for a little while.

As health and fitness became more central in my life, the buzz and escape weren't necessary anymore. Workouts, fitness, and hard-core exercise are my buzz. Being ripped and strong gives me my courage. Cardiovascular exercise brings peace of mind and relaxation now. I don't need some elixir or potion to help me escape anymore. If there's something amiss in my world, I get busy conquering it, not escaping from it.

When you're trying to lose weight, I don't recommend drinking alcohol at all, because alcohol suppresses fat oxidation and adds unnecessary calories to your diet, which either displace nutritious calories or erase your caloric deficit. I'm not here to tell you to stop drinking. If your doctor tells you that a glass of red wine at night is good for your heart, that's fine. But I can say confidently that alcohol will impede your progress during this 30-day plan. For the cleanse component to work, you need to phase out alcohol. I think you'll love what omitting spirits does for your mind, body, and spirit.

Tips on Transitioning Away from Alcohol

1. Anticipate all of the circumstances in which you would normally drink alcohol, and plan how to handle those situations. Either commit to saying no or find substitutes, such as sparkling water with a lemon or lime wedge.

2. If in the past you relied on alcohol to ease stress at the end of the day, plan to exercise at that time instead.

3. Find nondrinking friends who share your interest in health and fitness.

4. Notice how you feel mentally and physically after eliminating alcohol from your routine. Trust me, that feeling is powerful enough to help you abstain.

5. Consider supplementing with the amino acid glutamine, 2 to 4 grams daily. Glutamine helps diminish alcohol cravings. Another helpful supplement if you are a heavy drinker is milk

thistle. This botanical, with its high phytochemical content, can help reduce the potentially toxic effects of alcohol on the liver. For the proper dosage, follow the manufacturer's recommendation. (For more information on supplementation, see Chapter 16.)

Caffeine

Although caffeine does contain antioxidants, too much of it can compromise weight control. Caffeine taxes your adrenal glands and releases cortisol, a stress hormone, in the body. Adrenal stress associated with elevated cortisol levels can cause some profound issues with metabolism and tendencies to store fat. Cortisol encourages the body to accumulate fat, especially around the middle, where it does the most harm. This increases the risk of heart disease, diabetes, and high blood pressure. A lot of people who drink caffeine cannot lose their extra belly fat due to the overrelease of cortisol. Cortisol also increases sugar cravings and dehydrates the body. Caffeine itself can affect your sleep patterns and promote acidity in the body, leading to all kind of ill effects, digestive issues, and disease down the road.

The health effects of caffeine have been debated for years, and I predict that plenty of people will disagree with my opinion. Try to kick your coffee habit for 30 days and note how it affects your mood, energy, sleep patterns, and stress levels. There's no agreed-upon universal truth about coffee, so give this a try and see what happens. Then make a decision about what's best for you after the 30 days are up. I guarantee you will find your natural energy, and you won't want to go back to drinking your morning cup!

Tips on Transitioning Away from Caffeine

1. Identify sources of caffeine in your diet so that you know what to cut out. Refer to the chart on page 216 to help you determine this.
2. It's better to go cold turkey than taper off. Here's why: It's just too tough to see the effects of eliminating caffeine from your diet if you're still consuming even small amounts.
3. In place of coffee, sip caffeine-free herbal teas.
4. Common side effects of caffeine withdrawal are headaches and irritability. Sticking to your exercise program will combat these side effects.
5. Drink even more water than usual to help flush your system, carry needed chemicals to your brain, and rehydrate your body to give you more energy.
6. Change your routine so you're no longer involved in the chain reaction of events that contributes to your bad habits. Instead of drinking coffee in the kitchen, try sipping tea in the living room. Take a walk during your coffee break. Even something as simple as sitting in a different chair and using a different cup can remind you of the changes you're trying to make.

Caffeine Content in Beverages and Over-the-Counter Medicines

COFFEES	SERVING SIZE	CAFFEINE (MG)
Coffeehouse brewed coffee	16 oz	150–320
Blended coffee beverage	9.5 oz	115
Coffee, generic brewed	8 oz	102–200
Espresso	2 oz	30–40
Coffee, generic instant	8 oz	27–173
Coffee, generic decaffeinated	8 oz	3–12

TEAS	SERVING SIZE	CAFFEINE (MG)
Chai tea latte	16 oz	100
Snapple, lemon (and diet version)	16 oz	42
Tea, brewed	8 oz	40–120
Arizona Iced Tea, black	16 oz	32
Nestea	12 oz	26
Snapple, Just Plain Unsweetened	16 oz	18
Arizona Iced Tea, green	16 oz	15

SOFT DRINKS	SERVING SIZE	CAFFEINE (MG)
Jolt Cola	12 oz	72
Mountain Dew MDX, regular or diet	12 oz	71
Coke Red, regular or diet	12 oz	54
Mountain Dew, regular or diet	12 oz	54
Pepsi One	12 oz	54
Mellow Yellow	12 oz	53
Diet Coke	12 oz	47
Tab	12 oz	46.5
Diet Dr Pepper	12 oz	44
Dr Pepper	12 oz	42

Pibb Xtra, Diet Mr. Pibb, Pibb Zero	12 oz	41
Pepsi	12 oz	38
Pepsi Lime, regular or diet	12 oz	38
Diet Pepsi	12 oz	36
Coca-Cola Classic	12 oz	35
Coke Cherry, regular or diet	12 oz	35
Coke Lime	12 oz	35
Coke Vanilla	12 oz	35
Coke Zero	12 oz	35
7-Up, regular or diet	12 oz	0
Mug Root Beer, regular or diet	12 oz	0
Sprite, regular or diet	12 oz	0

ENERGY DRINKS	SERVING SIZE	CAFFEINE (MG)
Monster Energy	16 oz	160
Full Throttle	16 oz	144
Rip It, all varieties	8 oz	100
Tab Energy	10.5 oz	95
SoBe No Fear	8 oz	83
Red Bull	8.3 oz	80
Red Bull Sugarfree	8.3 oz	80
Rockstar Energy Drink	8 oz	80
SoBe Adrenaline Rush	8.3 oz	79
SoBe Essential Energy, berry or orange	8 oz	48

OVER-THE-COUNTER DRUGS	DOSAGE	CAFFEINE (MG)
No-Doz (Maximum Strength)	1 tablet	200
Vivarin	1 tablet	200
Excedrin (Extra Strength)	2 tablets	130
Anacin (Maximum Strength)	2 tablets	64

SOURCE: INFORMATION WAS OBTAINED FROM COMPANY WEB SITES AND THE CENTER FOR SCIENCE IN THE PUBLIC INTEREST.

Sugar

Man oh man, I love sugar! Homemade sweet things that contain deep dark chocolate make me weep. Sugar is my weakness, so if cutting it out completely sounds impossible to you, I can relate. But the fact is, candy, fruit juice, soda, and other processed foods that contain refined sugar are very rough on the body. Eaten in excess, it elevates heart-damaging triglycerides, adversely affects concentrations of heart-protective HDL cholesterol, contributes to yeast overgrowth in the body, causes weight gain, clouds your brain, and robs your body of important B vitamins.

Taking in a lot of sugar in a short period of time (or missing meals and then consuming sugar) can result in blood sugar spikes followed by hypoglycemia (low blood sugar). Hypoglycemia is marked by headaches, dizziness, anxiety, trembling, and irritability.

Food and Drinks Can Make You Fat and Rot Your Teeth

If you're trying to slim down, should you switch out your favorite sugary foods for "light" or "diet" varieties made with an artificial sweetener? Turns out, maybe not. According to some recent studies, consuming the fake stuff may lead to overeating. Research on this topic is relatively new—and so far, most of the testing has been done on animals. One study tested the weights of lab animals that were fed "light" yogurt containing saccharin versus those fed the traditional sugar-sweetened variety. The animals that were given yogurt sweetened with saccharin consumed more calories and packed on more pounds than the animals that were given the yogurt with sugar added. Why is this? Researchers believe that like humans', animals' brains are conditioned to expect sweet-tasting foods to be high in calories. When that no-calorie substitute is consumed instead, it seems to put the brain and the body in conflict. The brain thinks, "Mmm, satisfyingly sweet." And the body insists, "Wait. This isn't working. I need more." There are already human studies that link diet soft drinks to excess weight.[3]

If you value your pearly whites, here's another reason to avoid sodas, diet or regular. Most carbonated soft drinks cause wear and tear on your tooth enamel like you wouldn't believe. Whether they're full of sugar or not, bubbly drinks have some impact on tooth enamel. Citrus-flavored sodas do the most damage, followed by colas. The only exception seems to be root beer, which only causes a slight impact on tooth enamel.

It's not just the sugars in sodas that are bad for your teeth, it's the acids, too. The total acid content of the soda (including types like citric, phosphoric, malic, and tartaric acids) affects how much damage your choppers take. Some experts advise that rinsing your mouth after consuming a soda can reduce the damage, but who does that?

High-sugar foods and beverages can lead to skyrocketing blood sugar levels, which shift insulin production into high gear. When this high-sugar/high-insulin cycle repeats frequently, cells become overwhelmed with blood sugar and stop accepting it, a condition known as insulin resistance. Weight gain, increased risk for heart disease, and type 2 diabetes are among the results.

In addition, sugar interferes with the action of fat-burning and fat-storing hormones. Because a sugar overload triggers the secretion of extra insulin, the insulin starts orchestrating the movement of fat from the bloodstream into fat cells for storage. Insulin halts glucagon (a hormone that opposes the action of insulin) from entering the bloodstream, and glucagon is responsible for unlocking fat stores. The net effect is the ready conversion of sugar to body fat. In fact, as much as 35 percent of the sugar we eat will be stored in the body as fat.

Our body does need a little sugar for fuel, but rather than get it from the sugar bowl or refined sweets, you can obtain what your body needs from a healthy, whole food diet. Sugar is naturally present in many foods, such as grains and fruits. That's the best way to get the little sugar your body requires. Additionally, both fruit and whole grains contain fiber, which helps stabilize blood sugar.

Tips on Transitioning Away from Sugar

1. Sugar is hiding everywhere, but if you stick to the foods suggested in this plan, you should have no problem avoiding it.

2. Avoid high-fructose corn syrup (HFCS), a sweetener dumped into many foods. Two articles published in a 2004 issue of the *American Journal of Clinical Nutrition* suggest that HFCS and products containing it may contribute to America's epidemic of obesity and type 2 diabetes. When scientists investigated our food consumption patterns over the past 35 years, they discovered that between 1970 and 1990, consumption of HFCS rose by 1,000 percent—a trend that parallels the rise in obesity.[1,2] Another alarming piece of recent research has revealed that pancreatic tumor cells use fructose to divide and proliferate. That's the latest word from a team of researchers at UCLA, who published their study in the journal *Cancer Research*.

   The researchers grew pancreatic cancer cells in lab dishes and fed them both glucose and fructose, and the cells used the fructose to proliferate. Although it's found naturally in fruits, fructose is also a component of HFCS. (See the chart on page 220 to understand the difference among these sweeteners.)

   All of this makes the practice of reading food labels very important. Always check labels for added fructose as well as HFCS, which lurks in many processed foods—including ketchup and other condiments, sauces, salad dressing, jams, peanut butter, meat products, and commercially produced desserts.

3. Beware of juices. Fruit juices—even unsweetened juices—contain fructose and should be consumed in moderation, if at all.

4. Ban sodas (including diet sodas) from your home. Consider switching to an alternative, such as sparkling water, herbal tea, or green tea. (Stick to home-brewed teas, since most commercially bottled tea is brimming with HFCS.)

5. If you have a sweet tooth, grab fresh fruit whenever you feel the urge for something sweet. Or eat naturally sweet vegetables, such as sweet potatoes or squash, to help curb sugar cravings.

6. Plan ahead when you dine out. When the waiter comes to take your dessert order, condition yourself to say, "I'll just have some herbal tea."

7. Stop eating "dead" foods: junk, fried, and fast foods, as well as processed carbs. They're loaded with sugar and other additives. The more live foods we eat (fruits and vegetables), the more alive we feel. The more dead foods we eat . . . well, you get the idea.

Sugar Primer

TYPE OF SUGAR	WHAT IT IS
Beet sugar	Sucrose produced from sugar beets
Brown sugar	White sugar covered with a film of molasses
Coconut sugar	A nutrient-dense, low-glycemic sugar made from the sap of coconut flowers
Corn syrup	A sweetener made of glucose and water; produced by processing cornstarch to yield glucose
Fructose	Also called fruit sugar; found in fruit, some vegetables, honey, sugar cane, sugar beets, and other plants
Glucose	A sugar used by all living cells for energy
High-fructose corn syrup (HFCS)	A man-made liquid sweetener used in foods and beverages; produced by processing cornstarch to yield glucose, then processing that glucose to produce a high percentage of fructose
Molasses	An end product of sugarcane refining
Raw sugar	Also called turbinado sugar; a partially refined sugar extracted from cane juice; usually processed further to yield refined sugar (sucrose) and molasses
Sucrose (table sugar)	Commonly known as sugar and table sugar; a chemical combination of glucose and fructose, refined from sugarcane or sugar beets

Gluten

Found in wheat and a few other grains, gluten is a gluey protein that holds together bread, crackers, pastries, and many other heavy processed carbohydrates. It is the second most prevalent food substance in Western civilization, after sugar. Normal digestion doesn't entirely break down gluten. Surviving pieces come in contact with the lining of the bowel and the molecules of the immune system there. That molecular encounter results in an immune overreaction, in which the protein pieces are recognized as foreign invaders and come under attack. As a result, the digestive tract becomes inflamed and loses its villi, which are tiny, fingerlike projections that normally provide a vast surface area for absorbing digested nutrients. All of this results in gluten intolerance—the inability to digest gluten. Severe cases might indicate celiac disease, an inherited immune disorder.

Gluten intolerance used to be an unfamiliar affliction, seemingly affecting only a handful of people. Now some estimates say that up to 3 million Americans—about 1 in 133 people—have some form of gluten intolerance. Some signs of a gluten sensitivity are gas, bloating, acne or skin disruptions, aching joints, and clogged nasal passages.

Gluten also causes an acidic environment in the body, which can lead to inflammation, headaches, acne, weight gain, and behavioral issues. If you experience any symptoms of a gluten intolerance, removing gluten from your diet can make all the difference in the world.

Tips for Transitioning Away from Gluten

1. For now, throw away everything in your kitchen that contains gluten. That includes wheat, barley, rye, triticale, kamut, spelt, couscous, and oats (unless they're certified gluten-free); anything with modified food starch, malt, and malt flavorings; textured vegetable protein; hydrolyzed vegetable proteins; and many kinds of soy sauce. Then stock up on some ready-made alternatives, like gluten-free breads and cereals, but watch out for added sugars! Just because it's gluten-free doesn't mean it's healthy.

2. Identify the major sources of gluten in your diet. Do you eat lots of pasta, sandwiches, crackers, and cereals, plus cakes, cookies, and other sweets? Then you're eating a lot of gluten. Find alternatives for your favorites, such as corn, rice, wild rice, millet, buckwheat, amaranth, and quinoa. See the chart on page 222 for a list of some common gluten-free foods.

3. Some foods have more or less gluten in them than others. Foods with small amounts of gluten may not trigger sensitivities, unless a person has celiac disease. People who are diagnosed with this disease must give up not only most grain-based foods but also soups, sauces, canned foods, and hundreds of other items. This is because manufacturers frequently add gluten to processed foods. People who are less sensitive to gluten can usually eat sprouted grain breads, because although these breads contain gluten, sprouted wheat is easier for the body to digest.

4. Read labels carefully. Any product that contains wheat also contains gluten. Allergen statements on labels make it easier to find foods that contain wheat (labeling laws require disclosure of wheat within products). Once you've established that a product has no wheat, then make sure it's also free of rye, barley, and malt flavoring.

5. Stick to whole, fresh, unprocessed foods, as my plan suggests, and you'll make your diet naturally gluten-free by default.

Common Gluten-Free Foods

FLOURS

Almond	Corn	Rice	Taro
Bean	Pea	Soy	
Brown rice	Potato	Tapioca	

GRAINS AND GRAIN PRODUCTS

Amaranth	Millet	Quinoa	Wild rice
Buckwheat	Polenta	Rice cakes/crackers	
Cornmeal	Popcorn (check	Rice, ground, long	
Corn tortillas	coating)	or short grain	

FRUITS

All fresh and dried

VEGETABLES

All	All legumes, fresh and dried

LEAN PROTEINS

Beef	Fish	Poultry	Shellfish

DAIRY

Eggs	Dairy substitutes (almond milk, rice milk, and soy milk)	Cheeses Yogurt

FATS

Vegetable oils	Other fats

OTHER

Any food labeled "gluten-free"	Cassava	Nuts	Seeds
Arrowroot	Corn starch	Sago	
	Herbs		

Animal Products

On average, Americans individually consume around 185 pounds of meat per year (namely, beef, chicken, pork, and turkey), according to the U.S. Department of Agriculture (USDA). Such a heavy emphasis on meat and dairy products (as well as processed foods) leaves the average American with a serious overabundance of acids in his or her belly. The constant processing of all those excess acids can eventually drain the body's nutrient reserves. Unfortunately, a steady diet of acid-forming foods takes its toll over time. It can leach calcium from your bones, resulting in a weakened skeleton, and trigger many degenerative diseases, from colitis to rheumatoid arthritis to heart disease. To function properly, cells need to be slightly alkaline. Cutting back on meat and animal products will help your body alkalize. An alkalized body is a healthy body, and an acidic body is not—which is one reason that giving your body a break from animal protein is important.

We've all heard over the years that we must eat meat to get our protein requirements, but numerous studies done over the last 40 years prove that the protein in animal products is not as easily digested or assimilated by the body as plant- and grain-based proteins are. In fact, the digestive system has to work three times harder to digest meat than it does to digest veggies, fruits, and grains. Animal protein also clogs up the digestive tract, where it remains for 72 hours, has zero fiber, and makes it hard for your body to do its natural thing: eliminate! So do yourself a favor and give your body a break for 30 days. Notice how you feel, and you may even find that at the end of those 30 days you do not crave meat anymore or even like the way it tastes. I was a vegetarian for 15 years and was able to maintain plenty of lean muscle mass and energy to work out while avoiding meat. I promise you'll get enough protein from eating veggies, leafy greens, beans and legumes, nuts, seeds, and grains. For proof, refer to the chart on page 224 to see how well vegetarian sources of protein stack up against animal sources.

My Top 10 Toxic Foods

1. Soda, diet and regular
2. Sports drinks
3. Artificial sweeteners of any kind
4. White flour
5. White sugar
6. White potatoes and rice
7. Caffeine
8. Fried foods
9. Gluten
10. Dairy, especially ice cream and cheese (both high in heart-clogging trans fatty acids)

Tips on Transitioning Away from Animal Products

1. Select and try a few new vegetarian dishes from Melissa Costello in the Recipes section (see page 262).

2. Make veggies the focus of your meals and pair them with grains for complete nutrition. Eat your fill of greens and low-calorie vegetables. When it comes to starchier selections, like corn and sweet potatoes, watch your portion sizes.

3. Try dairy substitutes such as almond, rice, coconut, or soy milk (unsweetened), in addition to soy-

Protein Values for Common Foods

PROTEIN SOURCE*	PROTEIN CONTENT (IN GRAMS)
Soybeans, raw	36.49
Oats—1 cup cooked	33.78
Chicken, broilers or fryers, light meat only, cooked, roasted	30.91
Turkey, breast, roasted	28.71
Lentils, raw	28.06
Whitefish, cooked, dry heat	26.69
Quinoa—1 cup cooked	26.20
Salmon, cooked, dry heat	25.72
Nuts, walnuts, black	24.35
Beef, ground, regular, broiled, medium	24.07
Black beans, raw	21.60
Lima beans, large, mature seeds, raw	21.46
Almonds	21.26
Pinto beans, raw	20.88
Flaxseed	19.50
Tempeh, cooked	18.19
Chickpeas (garbanzo beans) boiled and drained—1 cup	17.72
Tofu, raw, firm	15.78
Lima beans, boiled and drained—1 cup	13.62
Egg, hard-boiled	12.58
Kidney beans, boiled and drained—1 cup	9.66

*EXCEPT WHERE NOTED, THE LISTINGS ARE BASED ON A 100-GRAM SERVING OF EACH (THE EQUIVALENT OF 3.53 OUNCES), LISTED IN DESCENDING ORDER FROM THE HIGHEST AMOUNT OF PROTEIN TO THE LOWEST AMOUNT OF PROTEIN. THE SOURCE OF THE DATA IS THE USDA NUTRIENT DATABASE.

based yogurts and cheeses. Try using dairy substitutes instead of milk in your favorite recipes. Your favorite dishes will turn out fine, and as an added bonus, you'll reduce the fat and cholesterol content.

4. Wake up to a delicious shake. Use soy milk and tofu along with your favorite fruit for a frothy high-protein smoothie to jump-start your day.

Enjoy the Results

My clients who have tried this 30-day plan say they are amazed at how quickly they see results after eliminating these five substances from their diets. Here's what Chuck and Susan told me.

Chuck's Story

As I come to the end of the 30 days, I have a ton of thoughts about what it has all meant to me. This plan is something I never would have thought I would take on. My mentality has always been: "Life is too short to deny yourself." But I promised to stick with it for the full 30 days.

Now I know how it feels to feel bad and how it feels to feel good. I also realize now that anything I set my mind to is possible. This is a very empowering feeling to experience.

The most common question I get is: "Chuck, are you going to eat meat and all the other stuff again?" Honestly, some of the things I will and some I will not, but I will hold true to the basics of nutrition: fruits, veggies, whole grains, healthy fats, and lean proteins. That being said, I did not do this cleanse to convert to a vegan lifestyle. That was not the purpose. It was a cleanse of my mind, body, and soul. For the most part, they are all sparkling clean, every part of me, and I feel great.

Susan's Story

Why would I subject myself to 30 days with no alcohol, sugar, caffeine, animal products (including fish, eggs, and dairy), or gluten? First of all, I have wanted to get off coffee for a while. I have been a two-, sometimes three-cupper a day for the past 20 years.

Second, I also was getting a little too attached to processed energy bars. Since I spend a lot of time taxiing my kids around town, I had gotten into this rut of grabbing a bar (or two) on my way out the door. Add a protein shake in there, and I realized that I was eating two bars and a shake a day and not enough whole foods.

So I decided to do this plan. One day turned into 2, then 3, and finally, by day 7, I started to feel like myself again. Not only that, I was starting to have more energy in the morning. I was waking up before my alarm and by the time I put my feet on the floor, I was wide awake and ready to hit the ground running.

I planned out all my meals for the entire week and made big batches of food that I could easily heat up or grab and eat in the car. After about 10 days, any cravings for sugar completely disappeared.

I feel amazing on this plan. I have more energy, I sleep better, I have less bloating (and all things relating to that), and I have clearer sinuses and skin. I usually get bad eczema on my arms in the winter, but so far, nothing. Someone in my Spin class told me my eyes seemed brighter. Not sure what that means, but heck, I'll take it!

So what happens on day 31? Well, I know I will not go back to coffee, except maybe an occasional decaf. I will not go back to dairy. I will probably add back fish and chicken as I do miss them, but probably not red meat. I will probably have an occasional drink every now and then. That leaves gluten and sugar. I am going to do my best to keep those to a minimum. My cravings have all but disappeared, and I feel amazing.

Cleanse Schedules for Beginners, Strivers, and Warriors

You do not have to eliminate all five substances at once; you'll do it slowly, following the guidelines below. Each level will phase out foods at a different pace and intensity. Beginners will phase out foods a little more gradually than Strivers or Warriors, for example. Follow the plan for your level.

Beginner's Instructions

Week 1: Eliminate coffee and caffeine-containing products (see page 216).

Week 2: Eliminate alcohol.

Week 3: Eliminate sugar and processed foods.

Week 4: Eliminate gluten-containing products.

After week 4: Eliminate dairy products one week and other animal products the next.

Striver's Instructions

Week 1: Eliminate coffee and caffeine-containing products (see page 216) and alcohol.

Week 2: Eliminate sugar and processed foods and gluten-containing products.

Week 3: Eliminate dairy products.

Week 4: Eliminate other animal products.

Warrior's Instructions

Week 1: Eliminate coffee and caffeine-containing products (see page 216), alcohol, and sugar and processed foods.

Week 2: Eliminate gluten-containing products.

Week 3: Eliminate dairy products.

Week 4: Eliminate other animal products.

I admit that it can be a challenge to make these changes, but if you take baby steps, you'll transform your habits into a healthier lifestyle that will stay with you for years to come.

Now that we've reviewed the Cleanse and the foods you won't be eating over the next 30 days, let's talk about the delicious foods you *will* be eating. Chapter 15 is all about nourishing your body with wholesome foods that fuel your workouts and make you feel good.

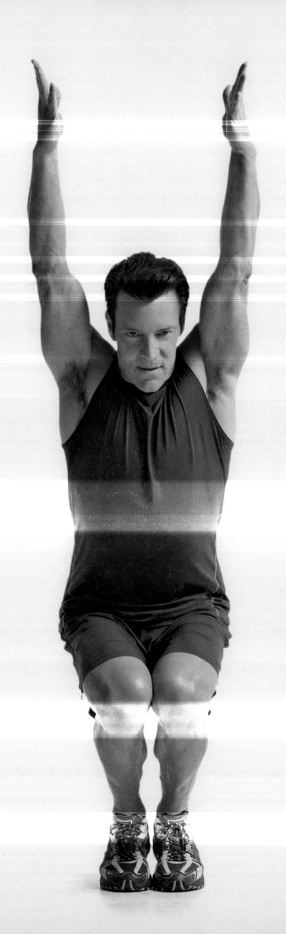

Part 2: Nourish

Here's where I show you the easy, convenient way to feel good and look good by eating the right foods so that you stay nourished with healthy food and nutrients and burn fat quickly. Now, don't worry; I'm not going to let you starve. My meal plan is a nourishing food plan that will keep you satisfied with delicious foods. What's more, it's a way of eating that you can live with for as long as you like. And it's simple. Eating right does not have to be convoluted.

Nourish

As you saw in the previous chapter, this plan is based on a powerful premise: What you eat has a direct effect on how you feel and how you look. Unhealthy processed foods tax our immune systems and organs, zap energy, and speed up the aging process. By contrast, healthy, whole foods fuel and heal us in a way that allows our bodies and our minds to do what we ask of them. These foods promote good digestion, better skin quality, improved muscle development, more energy, and enhanced mental well-being. In short, the right foods can give you a great body, great health, and a great outlook on life.

Here are the details of what you'll eat over the next 30 days (and beyond, hopefully).

What to Eat: Fantastic Fitness Foods

Leafy Greens (Serving size: unlimited; daily servings: unlimited)

Stock up on plenty of leafy greens, which are rich in minerals, micronutrients, vitamins, iron, and phytochemicals. Try some curly leaf kale or sauté some fresh spinach with garlic and olive oil. Your taste buds and your body will thank you! The following leafy greens are rich in disease-fighting micronutrients.

Arugula	Dandelion greens	Radicchio
Beet greens	Endive	Spinach
Bok choy	Kale	Turnip greens
Cabbage, all varieties	Lettuce, all varieties	Watercress
Chard	Mustard greens	
Collard greens	Parsley	

Vegetables (serving size: 1 cup, cooked or raw; daily servings: two or three)

Do you get your veggies out of a can or a freezer bag? Most canned vegetables have little nutritional value due to overprocessing, and most also contain a hefty dose of sodium. Always opt for fresh, organic vegetables when you can. If you are unable to buy fresh veggies, go with frozen. Most frozen vegetables retain the majority of their nutritional value and do not contain sodium. The following veggies will fill you up and give you a lot of energy for very few calories.

Alfalfa	Eggplant	Radishes
Artichokes	Fennel	Rhubarb
Artichoke hearts	Green beans	Rutabaga
Asparagus	Jicama	Scallions
Beets	Leeks	Summer squash
Broccoli	Kohlrabi	Sweet potatoes
Broccoli sprouts	Mushrooms	Swiss chard
Brussels sprouts	Okra	Tomatoes
Carrots	Onion	Turnips
Cauliflower	Parsnips	Winter squash (acorn, butternut, etc.)
Celery	Pea pods	
Chile peppers	Peppers, all varieties	Yams
Corn	Potatoes	Yellow wax beans
Cucumbers	Pumpkin	Zucchini

Legumes (serving size: 1 cup cooked, except as noted below; *weekly* servings: four or five)

I believe that legumes are a near-perfect food. Not only are they loaded with protein, fiber, and vitamins, but they're also inexpensive and so easy to add to any meal. Use the following options in soups, salads, and dips or as a source of vegetarian protein in place of meat.

Adzuki beans	Great Northern beans	Peas
Black beans	Hummus (½ cup)	Pinto beans
Black-eyed peas	Kidney beans	Red beans
Broad beans	Lentils	Soybeans
Chickpeas	Lima beans	Split peas
Fava beans	Navy beans	White beans

Fruits (serving size: one whole fruit or 1 cup fresh berries or chopped fresh fruit, except as noted below; daily servings: two or three)

I can't say it too many times or in too many different ways: Nothing beats fresh fruit. After all, it comes packed with vitamins, minerals, and phytochemicals. For the most nutrition, eat fruit fresh and raw, and leave the skin on whenever possible. Most fruits and vegetables carry the majority of their antioxidants (and fiber) in their skins—so don't peel them! Always wash fruit well in warm water, and choose organic fruits whenever possible. The following superfruits are not only delicious, but they'll also help support a healthy immune system and keep you energized all day.

Apples	Grapefruit (½ fruit)	Plums
Apricots (2)	Guava	Pomegranates
Bananas	Honeydew	Prunes
Blackberries	(¼ melon)	Raisins
Blueberries	Lemons	Raspberries
Cantaloupe	Limes	Strawberries
(¼ melon)	Mangoes	Tangelos
Casaba (¼ melon)	Oranges	Tangerines
Cherries	Papayas	Watermelon
Cranberries	Peaches	(large wedge)
Figs (2)	Pears	Virtually any
Grapes	Pineapple	fresh fruit
Kiwifruit (2)	(1 cup chopped	
Kumquats (2)	fresh fruit)	

Whole Grains (serving size: ½ cup cooked, except as noted below; daily servings: two or three)

Whole grains, like those listed below, are the quintessential health food, supplying high-quality complex carbohydrates, protein, fat, fiber, and a host of micronutrients in an easy-to-prepare package that also happens to taste good. Whole grains are low in saturated fat and provide a good dose of soluble fiber, which can absorb excess cholesterol and aid in shuttling it out of the body, helping to keep arteries clear. Soluble fiber also helps stabilize blood sugar levels, which is why eating soluble fiber–rich grains, such as oatmeal, seems to improve insulin sensitivity and may help ward off type 2 diabetes. But that's not all. Whole grains supply lots of antioxidants that may offer disease protection.

High-fiber whole grain foods are also slimming. According to a study published in the *American Journal of Clinical Nutrition*, when dieters ate four or five servings of whole-grain foods daily for 12 weeks, they lost a significantly higher percentage of fat (including in their midsection) than those who ate only refined grains.[1] One theory is that insoluble fiber, also found in whole grains, makes you feel full faster by slowing your digestion, so you eat fewer calories.

Here's a list of my favorite whole grains.

Barley

Brown rice, long grain

Brown rice, short grain

Gluten-free pasta

Oats, preferably steel cut and gluten-free

Rice crackers or gluten-free crackers (4 crackers = 1 serving)

Sprouted-grain bread (1 slice = 1 serving)

Wild rice

Pseudograins (serving size: ½ cup cooked; daily servings: two or three)

Technically, the grains listed below are considered pseudograins, meaning they do not belong to the grass family. However, most health experts still consider them whole grains because they share a similar nutritional profile and offer the same health benefits as whole grains do.

Amaranth

Millet

Quinoa

Soy-Based Proteins (serving size: ½ cup; *weekly* servings: one or two)

If you've never tried the proteins listed below, now is a great time to do so. Tofu is made by coagulating soy milk and pressing the resulting curds into blocks. Packages of tofu read "extra firm," "firm," "soft," and "silken." The descriptions are an indication of the amount of water in the cube. Tempeh is an Indonesian diet staple made from whole, cooked soybeans that are cultured and fermented. It has a nutty, chewy flavor. Both tofu and tempeh (as well as all soy foods) have numerous health benefits, such as strengthening bones, lowering cholesterol levels, and possibly even preventing stroke, heart disease, and cancer.

A word of caution: Go easy on soy foods. Too much soy in the diet may cause mineral deficiencies. It may hinder calcium absorption, for example. What's more, excessive amounts of soy may lead to thyroid problems. If you like soy, enjoy it in moderation—once or twice a week.

Tempeh

Tofu

Lean Proteins (serving size: one palm-size portion; daily servings: up to two)

During the weeks that you eat animal-based protein, try to select organic, free-range, wild-caught, or grass-fed products to ensure the best nutrition. Choose grass-fed beef; it has less fat and more health-protective omega-3 fatty acids than nonorganic beef. Look at the color: The deeper the red, the leaner the meat. For the leanest cuts of meat, look for loin or round in the name, such as sirloin and eye of round.

You'll notice that shellfish is included in my list of healthy seafood options. Although doctors used to advise patients with elevated cholesterol to avoid consumption of shellfish, the latest research shows that moderate shellfish consumption is beneficial to patients with cholesterol problems. A study published in the *American Journal of Clinical Nutrition* revealed the following: Oyster, clam, crab, and mussel diets lowered triglycerides (potentially dangerous blood fats) and overall cholesterol. And oysters and mussels improved HDL cholesterol (the beneficial kind).[2]

One reason is that shellfish is generally high in omega-3 fatty acids and monounsaturated fats. Both increase your HDL level and decrease your LDL level, as well as help reduce levels of triglycerides in your blood.

SEAFOOD	Monkfish	Scallops
Clams	Orange roughy	Shark
Cod	Oysters	Shrimp
Flounder	Perch	Sole
Grouper	Pollock	Tilapia
Haddock	Red snapper	Trout
Halibut	Salmon, wild	Tuna (fresh or low-sodium canned)
Lobster	Sardines,	
Mackerel	water-packed	Whitefish

Lean Proteins, continued

EGGS AND POULTRY

Chicken breast, skinless

Cornish hen, skinless

Egg (1)

Egg whites (2)

Turkey breast, skinless

LEAN MEATS

Eye of round

Ground beef with
    less than 10% fat

Tenderloin

Top loin

Top round

Top sirloin

Dairy and Dairy Substitutes (serving size: 8 ounces or 1 cup, or 1 ounce hard soy-based cheese—other serving sizes noted below; daily servings: up to two)

You'll be scaling back on dairy while following my plan, so I want to give you a pep talk on dairy substitutes. A lot of people don't get along well with cow's milk because they're lactose intolerant, meaning they lack an enzyme needed to digest lactose, the sugar in milk. Some people want to cut back on their intake of saturated fat and cholesterol, and others are still trying to give up that last shred of animal product in their diets. Fortunately, there are many great-tasting dairy alternatives on the market that serve as fine substitutes.

As for cheeses, look for those made from sheep's or goat's milk; they're easier to digest than cow's milk cheese. Even people who claim to be lactose intolerant can usually handle these types of cheeses. I encourage you to try the following healthy dairy and nondairy foods.

REGULAR DAIRY

Low-fat and fat-free
    milk, organic

Low-fat yogurt,
    organic

Sheep's or goat's milk
    cheeses

DAIRY SUBSTITUTES

Almond milk

Coconut milk

Rice milk

Soy milk

Soy-based cheeses

Soy-based yogurt

Seeds (serving size: 1 tablespoon; *weekly* servings: two or three)

Snack on seeds or sprinkle them over salads; you can also soak seeds in water to soften them before mixing them into smoothies or soup. (But avoid boiling liquids—the seeds' fatty acids break down at high heat.) Seeds are perishable and can easily turn rancid, so be sure to store them in the fridge.

You'll notice chia seeds on the list below. Yes, they're better known as the main ingredient of the Chia Pet (the once-popular sprouting animal figurine), but they are surprisingly nutritious. Full of antioxidants, calcium, potassium, magnesium, iron, and zinc, just 2 tablespoons contain 6 grams of omega-3s, 10 grams of fiber, and 7 grams of protein.

As for flaxseed, it's an excellent source of omega-3 fatty acids, lignans (phytochemicals thought to fight cancer and diabetes), fiber, and protein.

Chia seeds

Flaxseed

Nuts (serving size: ¼ cup; *weekly* servings: two or three)

Most nuts are great sources of monounsaturated fats, now recognized as some of the most beneficial fats you can eat. Many of them can help lower artery-clogging LDL cholesterol levels. Some, such as Brazil nuts and almonds, contain important antioxidants. And all of them are rich in a spectrum of nutrients, including magnesium, manganese, vitamin E, and healthful compounds, such as phytosterols—plant lipids that decrease the body's absorption of cholesterol and may have some cancer-preventing effects. More good news: Eating a handful of raw nuts before a meal can keep your appetite under control. Here are some of my favorites.

Almonds

Brazil nuts

Cashews

Hazelnuts

Pecans

Healthy Fats (serving size: 2 tablespoons oils or ¼ of an avocado; daily servings: one)

Everyone needs fat for energy. But not all fats are created equal, so be sure to choose healthy fats like those listed below. Limit saturated fats, including cream and butter, which come from animals, as well as trans fatty acids—the artery-clogging result of turning oils into room-temperature solids. You can cook with any of the oils listed below; they are stable at high temperatures.

Almond oil

Avocado

Coconut oil, extra virgin

Flaxseed oil

Olive oil, extra virgin

Walnut oil

Creating Your Meals

Now that you know what foods you'll be eating, let's look at how you can build them into a 7-day meal plan. This example incorporates several of the delicious dishes you'll find in the Recipes section (see page 262).

Monday

Breakfast: Egg white omelet with fresh veggies and avocado or *Tony's Power Protein Smoothie* (page 263); peach or other seasonal fruit

Snack: Apple with 1 tablespoon nut butter

Lunch: *Lentil Soup* (page 269) with tossed green salad and *Lemon Vinaigrette* (page 272)

Snack: Hummus with sliced cucumbers and rice crackers

Dinner: *Gingery Vegetable Stir-Fry* (page 280) with tempeh or chicken breast over quinoa

Tuesday

Breakfast: Two whole grain waffles with 1 tablespoon nut butter and drizzled with agave syrup; ½ grapefruit

Snack: Hard-boiled egg; 1 tablespoon hummus

Lunch: *Divine Rice Wrap* (page 281) with *Quinoa Black Bean Salad with Dried Apricots* (page 273)

Snack: Piece of fresh fruit with ½ ounce raw nuts

Dinner: *Fresh Pesto, Tomato, and Zucchini Pasta* (page 274); *Raw Spinach Salad with Fennel* (page 271)

Coconut Oil: Is It the Ultimate Fat?

Coconut oil has gotten a bad rap in the past, but researchers are discovering new evidence that suggests it may actually be much healthier than we thought. Coconut oil contains compounds responsible for many of its unique benefits. The oil boasts lauric acid (also found in mother's milk), which helps kill harmful bacteria and viruses. Caprylic acid, also found in coconut oil, is thought to be a potent antifungal agent and may hold promise for treating athlete's foot, *Candida,* and other fungal conditions.

One of the most exciting properties of coconut oil is its fat-burning power. The credit goes to the oil's concentration of medium-chain triglycerides (MCTs), which appear to be digested differently than other fats. Instead of being packed away into fat cells, MCTs are used to produce energy. This boost in energy production stimulates metabolism.

Soup: It's What's for Breakfast!

I have been known to eat soup for breakfast, and I'm pretty sure there must be a federal law against that. Seriously though, should soup be reserved only for lunch or dinner? A restorative bowl of soup for breakfast, by the way, is traditional in many parts of the world.

So why not turn the table, so to speak, and start your day with soup? Soup is nutritious, delicious, and filling. It just makes sense as a morning meal. Instead of confining certain foods to certain meals, let's be flexible. Oatmeal and grapefruit for dinner, anyone?

Wednesday

Breakfast: *Melissa's Roasted Butternut Squash Soup* (page 268) with ¼ cup cooked brown rice or quinoa mixed in

Snack: Green apple with 1 tablespoon nut butter

Lunch: *Kitchen Sink Veggie Soup* (page 267); *Brussels Sprouts Salad with Cranberries and Almonds* (page 272)

Snack: Crackers with bruschetta; ¼ of a melon

Dinner: Salmon with quinoa and broccoli

Thursday

Breakfast: One piece of sprouted-grain toast with 1 tablespoon nut butter and ½ banana

Snack: Piece of fresh fruit with ½ ounce raw nuts

Lunch: *Supreme Vegetarian Burrito* (page 279) with tossed green salad; 1 apple

Snack: 1 cup *Warm Artichoke and Chickpea Salad* (page 271)

Dinner: *Baked Apricot-Glazed Chicken Breasts* (page 282) with *Lemon Garlic Green Beans* (page 275) and cooked brown rice

Friday

Breakfast: Steel-cut oats with almond milk and a fistful of fresh berries

Snack: Edamame with sea salt

Lunch: Green salad with veggies, seeds, and a veggie burger on top; 1 orange

Snack: 1 cup vegetarian vegetable soup

Dinner: Salmon with quinoa and *Raw Spinach Salad with Fennel* (page 271)

Saturday

Breakfast: Sprouted-grain English muffin with 1 tablespoon nut butter; 1 cup fresh berries

Snack: Carrots and cucumber slices with hummus

Lunch: *Supreme Vegetarian Burrito* (page 279) with tossed green salad and *Lemon Vinaigrette* (page 272)

Snack: Hard-boiled egg with crackers; or *Tony's Power Protein Smoothie* (page 263)

Dinner: *Gingery Vegetable Stir-Fry* (page 280) with tempeh over brown rice and *Raw Spinach Salad with Fennel* (page 271)

Sunday

Breakfast: Coconut yogurt with fresh berries, almonds, and an apple

Snack: *Melissa's "Cheesy" Popcorn* (page 265)

Lunch: *Black Bean Yam Chili* (page 276) with tossed green salad; one piece of fresh fruit

Snack: *Oven-Baked Yam Chili "Fries"* (page 275) with fruit-sweetened ketchup

Dinner: Large green salad with veggies, seeds, and a veggie burger on top

The Calorie Question

When it comes to food, I have never been a calorie counter—I have enough things to think about, and tracking my calories is not one of them. But it is important to be aware of calories. The simple truth about achieving a healthy weight boils down to getting fit and burning more calories than you consume during the day. If you follow this plan faithfully, exercise included, you won't have to worry about counting calories because you'll be incinerating them automatically.

I'm equally uninterested in percentages, formulas, and strange food combinations that supposedly trick the body into losing weight for a short period of time. This battle of overeating, eating garbage pretending to be food, and dangerous weight loss adds up to very short-term gains. If you really care about your health and want to stay fit for years to come, then you must clean up your diet so that your mind and body run smoothly.

Eating Out: Ask for What You Need

I've never been to a restaurant where I couldn't get what I wanted for a healthy meal. Fried fish joints, steak houses, fast-food emporiums—you name it, I've been there and I've eaten nutritiously.

The secret is simple: Ask for what you need, and 95 percent of the time you will get it, because restaurants want your business and waiters want tips. Here's how to ask.

"I'm on a special diet [or "I'm allergic to a certain food"]. Is it okay if we create something from scratch?" Let's say you see fish on the menu. Ask to have it grilled or at least not swimming in butter. Or if you're at an Italian restaurant, ask for a half portion of pasta with lots of veggies and some marinara sauce. Do that and you've got a superhealthy meal.

I was at a steak restaurant recently, and since I don't eat red meat, I ordered wild salmon. I skipped down to the bottom of the menu and noticed there were à la carte vegetables. I ordered side dishes of broccoli, spinach, and asparagus. So I had a nice piece of salmon with three vegetables surrounding it. I was the happiest guy in the place.

Here are some additional guidelines.

1. *Ask* that bread not be brought to your table.
2. *Ask* about preparation methods.
3. *Ask* for a take-home container at the beginning of your meal, and fill it with any food on your plate that exceeds one portion size. One protein serving is about the size of the palm of your hand. One serving of rice is about as big as your fist.
4. *Ask* that salad dressing be served on the side so you can control the amount you consume. Add the dressing sparingly, or dip the salad into the dressing before each bite.
5. *Ask* for plain, unbuttered vegetables with any special sauces (hollandaise, cheese, or lemon butter) on the side.
6. When getting together with a group, *ask* if everyone would try out an ethnic restaurant (the more authentic the better). Japanese, Greek, Middle Eastern, African, and Indian restaurants all generally provide vegetarian options.

Guidelines for Success

Here are some essential guidelines to follow as you begin your new eating plan.

1. Drink at least eight glasses of water daily in addition to other liquids (like caffeine-free herbal tea). Thirst often masquerades as hunger. Keep a bottle or glass of water on your desk and sip it throughout the day.
2. Avoid margarine, hydrogenated oils, and fat substitutes.
3. Eat more fresh foods than frozen or canned products. Buy seasonal and local produce, which provide the highest nutrient value at the lowest price. Eating seasonally balances the body and provides proper nutrition. And save money by buying in bulk seasonally—fruits, grains, beans, nuts, seeds, and so forth.

4. Steer clear of artificial sweeteners. Chemical sweeteners have no calories and no nutritive value. Research suggests that when you eat or drink foods containing these sweeteners, your body interprets the sweetness as a sign that more food is on the way. Drinking diet soda, for example, can increase your desire for sweet flavors, which may lead you to eat more sweet nonnutritive foods.

5. Use agave nectar to sweeten foods. Made from the juice of the Mexican blue agave plant, agave nectar is a honeylike substance that contains 60 calories per tablespoon. You need less of it to achieve the same level of sweetness you'd get from sugar: In most recipes, you can substitute ¼ cup of agave for 1 cup of sugar. Our bodies digest agave nectar slowly, so our blood sugar and insulin levels don't undergo the dramatic spike that occurs when we eat sugar. Agave also contains beneficial minerals, including calcium, iron, magnesium, and potassium.

6. Stick to your recommended foods as closely as you can.

7. Eat a variety of foods every day.

8. Don't skip breakfast. Breakfast really is the most important meal of the day. Eating a healthy, well-balanced meal in the morning helps you sustain your energy levels and can prevent those late-day sugar/carb snack cravings that are many people's downfall.

9. Try the recipes beginning on page 262. They are easy to follow, simple to prepare, and tasty.

10. Cook in bulk. Spend some time in the kitchen on the weekend and prepare a full week's worth of food. Divide big batches of meals like chili or soup into individual serving sizes and store them in the fridge or freezer for easy weeknight meals.

11. Practice "conscious eating"—eat slowly and savor every bite. Eating consciously gives your brain time to catch up with your stomach so that you're aware of being full. You'll know when you've had just enough food to be satisfied.

12. Commit to the full 30 days. Afterward, note how you feel. Based on that self-evaluation, decide which foods you will forgo permanently, which foods you will limit, and which foods you will add back in and eat moderately.

13. Finally, don't try to buck the plan by getting caught up in fad diets and weight-loss potions. Long-term success happens when you consistently exercise and eat healthy foods. Our bodies don't run on exercise; they run on the fuel we put in our mouths. Good diet and exercise have to happen at the same time, however. If you bring the same level of consistency and discipline to your daily fuel intake as you do to your workouts, you'll greatly reduce a lifetime of health risks, improve your overall quality of life, and see much greater physical changes in a shorter period of time.

Love the Benefits!

Based on what I've observed from my clients and the mail I've received from people who use my programs, you should begin to see weight loss within the first week or so. It's common to lose up to 3 to 5 pounds in the first week.

Don't be surprised if your cholesterol levels improve as well, although this may take up to 10 weeks. I've talked to people on cholesterol-lowering drugs who were able to reduce their doses or even go off them, but let your doctor guide you.

If you have high blood pressure, it may improve gradually, too. The positive effects of eating more fruits and vegetables (many of which contain potassium) really add up.

And there are other benefits to including more whole foods in your diet. If you are bothered by occasional constipation, you will probably find that you become more regular. People with type 2 diabetes may see their blood sugar levels improve. Your skin will be clearer, not to mention younger looking. And almost everyone reports feeling healthier and more energetic overall. There's nothing to lose—except ugly fat and bad health habits!

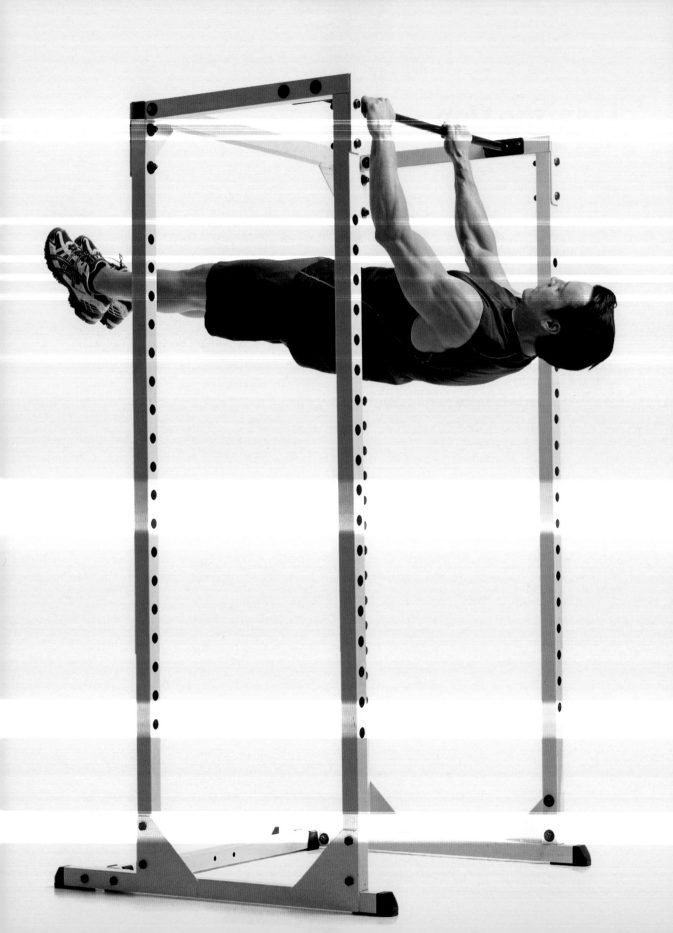

16

Part 3: Supplement

I get asked all of the time about the supplements I take. People want to know if they need to take supplements to get ripped, which ones I recommend, and whether or not supplementation is safe.

I will answer all of these questions and more, but let me start by saying that I believe strongly in nutritional supplementation. I have an entire kitchen cabinet devoted to supplements. I take them in the morning, and I take them at night. What I know is this: If I miss even 2 days of taking my supplements, I don't feel as energetic. I don't recover from workouts as quickly. A little tendinitis in my elbow or knee might flare up. My mental processes fog over like a windshield on a damp day. There's a clear cause and effect here: When I take supplements, I feel good. When I don't take them, I feel like crap. So I take my supplements every day, at home and on the road. My belief is that going without them is like going without water. I couldn't be the athlete I am today without them.

Supplements perform two vital functions: (1) They help you recover from the workouts, and (2) they supply the nutrients your body needs to heal and be healthy. Think about it: Several times a week, you are putting your body through a grueling workout of plyometrics, resistance training, yoga, and more. As a consequence, energy-giving glycogen stores are depleted; muscle protein is dismantled; microscopic tears in muscle fibers occur; energy-producing compounds are lost from cells; fluid and electrolytes dwindle; and disease-causing free radicals proliferate. Your body is then thirsting for "recovery," the process of regeneration that takes place in the aftermath of a workout. You need to supply your body with all the nutritional building blocks it needs to restore what's lost and repair what's damaged. The benefits of doing this are numerous: greater energy levels each time you exercise, less fatigue, increased muscular development, and stronger immunity so you don't have to miss workouts. Supplementing your diet with the proper nutrients, such as carbs, electrolytes, antioxidants, and more, can aid the recovery process.

Taking supplements may be one of the healthiest habits you can adopt. Mounting research suggests that supplements can help protect you against diseases like heart disease and cancer, plus maintain healthy bones, muscles, and joints. Supplementation and eating well also reduce bouts of depression, sadness, and anxiety, while promoting psychological well-being.

In a perfect world, we'd get all the nutrients we need on our dinner plates. But in the real world, most of us don't even come close. In fact, less than one-fourth of us eat the five daily servings of fruits and vegetables recommended by the American Heart Association. Factor in a national fondness for refined flour and sugar, and we're pretty much guaranteed to fall short of the nutritional mark. Even "enriched" flour is only augmented with some of the nutrients (the B vitamins) that were lost in the refining process, while refined sugar contains no vitamins or minerals at all. Because poor-quality food is so rampant these days, supplementation is more important than ever. Even if you are following my meal plan and making healthy choices, I still believe that supplementation will provide a needed boost to your workouts and your health.

Supplements versus Drugs

Every day, millions of Americans fumble through their medicine chests searching for pills, both over-the-counter and prescription, to make their symptoms go away. But by and large, most drugs simply mask pain and symptoms without curing the underlying cause of a condition. Supplements, on the other hand, work with your body to heal the cause of the problem. Supplements generally take longer to yield results, but they may provide a gentler path to healing. I am not saying you should give up any prescription written by a doctor. Pharmaceutical drugs provide a vital defense against infections and help us survive many serious diseases.

If you decide to ask your physician about restocking your medicine chest, there are some supplemental alternatives that could help control the most common types of distress. If you suffer from migraines, for example, you may find relief by taking a magnesium supplement. Glucosamine and chondroitin are often recommended for osteoarthritis pain and stiffness, which is caused by loss of cartilage in the joint. A dozen studies have shown that these supplements reduce the symptoms of osteoarthritis by about 40 percent, on average. Garlic may help control high cholesterol that's the result of consuming too many fatty and sugary foods. Turmeric helps with digestion, as well as with inflammation and pain. My advice—and I'm sure you've heard this umpteen times before—is to check with your doctor before taking any supplements.

What Supplements Do You Need?

Everyone is different. Age, weight, stress, gender, exercise intensity—all of these things factor in to which supplements are important. At certain life stages many people require more of particular nutrients than their diet can provide, such as folic acid for women of childbearing age or calcium for pregnant and nursing women. And I'm sure you know that boning up on calcium may help some women stave off the brittle bone disease, osteoporosis. Calcium, combined with other nutrients, may also help to protect against colon cancer.

The Supplement Component: My Super 11 Supplement Program

In the next few pages I'll give you a rundown of the supplements I take and recommend. Then you can judge for yourself whether supplements should be a part of your overall wellness plan. Here goes.

1. Multivitamin/Multimineral

Why You Might Need This: Even if you eat a balanced diet, I think you should consider taking a multivitamin and a multimineral. Even the most healthful diets may still lack the necessary levels of vitamins and minerals. Few doctors and health professionals would disagree. In fact, several years ago, an influential study reported in the *Journal of the American Medical Association (JAMA)* suggested that all adults should take a daily multivitamin to prevent chronic diseases like cancer and heart disease. The report, written by researchers and physicians at Harvard Medical School, was based on a review of 152 studies published during the past 40 years. Most experts agree that any multi containing 100 percent of the recommended requirements for each nutrient is adequate.[1]

If your multi is an antioxidant formula, all the better. An essential part of recovery involves mustering your body's antioxidant defense forces. When you exercise, there's a dramatic increase in the amount of oxygen used by your body. A fraction of this oxygen is converted into free radicals, which are unstable oxygen molecules that attack body tissues. Normally, free radicals are not a big problem. But during strenuous activity, free radicals can start outnumbering antioxidants—a condition called oxidative stress. This may leave you vulnerable to disease.

Plus, when you damage muscle cells during exercise, your body is left with a lot of debris for your immune cells to clean up. Think of this scenario as equivalent to a group of janitors arriving to clean up a mess. They get help from antioxidant vitamins like E and C. In short, antioxidants will help repair and clean up the rubbish left over from torn-up muscle fibers—and that, my friends, is crucial.

The Calcium Conundrum

There is a great deal of confusion and controversy about which form of calcium is best. Some women suffer from constipation, nausea, and indigestion with calcium supplementation, especially from calcium carbonate. Calcium citrate is less likely to cause these problems. Calcium carbonate is absorbed well when taken with food. Calcium citrate can be taken with food, but when taken on an empty stomach, it is absorbed better than calcium carbonate. And calcium citrate may be a better choice for older women whose lower stomach acid production and lower intake of vitamin D—due to less exposure to sunshine and decreased fat absorption—compromise optimal calcium absorption. Some research suggests that combining calcium citrate with vitamin D_3 allows it to be more easily absorbed. Best advice: Talk to your doctor about which form is best for you.

Effective Dosage: Follow the manufacturer's recommendations. Because vitamins and minerals are particles of food, it's best to take them with food for maximum uptake by your body.

Note: If you are a woman over age 50, it's unlikely that your multivitamin will contain sufficient levels of magnesium and calcium to meet your needs. Seek out a separate calcium-magnesium supplement with at least 100 milligrams of magnesium and 1,000 milligrams of calcium.

2. B-Complex

Why You Might Need This: B-complex vitamins help convert food into energy; help the nervous system and brain function at optimal levels; aid stress relief; maintain healthy skin, eyes, and hair; promote muscle tone in the gastrointestinal tract; and support the immune system. B vitamins are easily flushed out of the body, and people on weight-loss diets, alcoholics, or those who take antibiotics or seizure drugs are even more inclined to have a vitamin B deficiency.

Effective Dosage: 50 to 300 milligrams daily. Formulas of B-complex vitamins typically provide all the B vitamins in the correct proportions. The Bs are water-soluble and pass through the body quickly, so take them in a time-release formula or divide up your dose and take it with food over the course of your day.

3. Vitamin C

Why You Might Need This: Vitamin C is a powerful antioxidant that slows aging, aids tissue repair, enhances immunity, helps you handle stress, maintains healthy gums, activates folic acid, and increases iron absorption.

Effective Dosage: 500 to 3,000 milligrams daily. Our bodies don't make vitamin C, so we need outside sources. Ester-C is the better form. It's nonacidic, enters the blood faster, and stays in tissues longer. (Combine it with bioflavonoids for a greater effect.) Vitamin C rapidly flushes away in urine, so take it in a time-release formula or divide up your dose and take it with food over the course of your day.

4. Fish Oil

Why You Might Need This: Fish oil contains omega-3 fatty acids, which help regulate the cardiovascular, reproductive, nervous, and immune systems; are a component of cell membranes; prevent blood clots; lower levels of triglycerides and cholesterol; reduce inflammation; promote healthy skin, hair, and nails; transport oxygen to the tissues; and lessen PMS and perimenopausal symptoms. Most doctors today recommend that we all supplement our diets with fish oil.

Effective Dosage: 250 to 3,000 milligrams daily. Divide up your dose and take it with food over the course of your day.

5. Ginkgo Biloba

Why You Might Need This: I've read up on this herb's effects on the brain. It is thought to improve circulation and thereby increase the flow of blood and nutrients to the brain. This may make it an especially useful memory-booster for middle-aged and older people, since blood flow to the brain diminishes as we age. Of course, there are studies that say ginkgo is all smoke and mirrors. All I know is that when I take it, I remember things, and when I don't, I'm forgetful.

Effective Dosage: Aim for 120 to 160 milligrams a day, divided into three doses.

6. Coenzyme Q$_{10}$

Why You Might Need This: Coenzyme Q$_{10}$ is an antioxidant and produces energy in every cell of your body. It also has anti-aging effects, increases tissue oxygenation, strengthens the heart muscle, treats angina and high blood pressure, reverses gum deterioration, aids circulation, and enhances immunity. It also may lower the risk of recurrent breast cancer.

Effective Dosage: 30 to 200 milligrams daily with food that contains fat. Gel capsules are more potent and more easily absorbed than powdered products.

7. Green Foods

Why You Might Need This: The term *green foods* generally refers to about half a dozen foods recognized as having the highest chlorophyll content: barley grass and other cereal grasses, wheat grass, alfalfa, spirulina, and chlorella. Chlorophyll, the pigment that gives plants their emerald hue, is the magical substance that makes greens so great. Chlorophyll is often compared to hemoglobin, the red coloring in blood that delivers oxygen to our trillions of cells. The notable difference between these two substances is that in the center of the chlorophyll molecule there is magnesium, while in the center of hemoglobin there is iron. Because of the similarities in their structures, scientists postulated that chlorophyll in plants could be effective in treating blood and circulation disorders, including anemia and high blood pressure, in humans.

Not only are green foods rich in chlorophyll, they also contain a spectrum of beneficial nutrients that are said to fight infection and remove toxins from the body. They're full of antioxidant vitamins, minerals, amino acids, and fiber. And they're loaded with active enzymes, generally in short supply in the typical refined-and-processed American diet. Because many of the brands on the market are spiked with other nutrients like mushrooms, carrots, beets, ginger, garlic, herbs, vitamins, and minerals, nutrient-dense green foods can fill in substantial nutritional blanks. It's sort of like having a salad in a glass.

Effective Dosage: Follow the manufacturer's recommendations. Most brands recommend a scoop or more of powder mixed with water or vegetable juice.

8. Red Foods

Why You Might Need This: I'm on the road a lot, so I don't always have access to fresh, organic fruit. In its place, I take a superconcentrated fruit powder that is naturally high in antioxidants, vitamins, minerals, and phytochemicals. This particular supplement is an extract of certain red foods—namely, cranberries, red grapes, watermelon, cherries, and tomatoes. These foods contain compounds that give deep red, purple, and blue hues to fruits and vegetables, and these substances may help protect our bodies against cancer, heart disease, and other life-threatening illnesses.

Effective Dosage: Follow the manufacturer's recommendations. These products typically come in capsules or powders you can mix with liquids.

9. Oregano Oil

Why You Might Need This: The flavor and fragrance of this popular herb are inextricably associated with its use in flavoring tomato dishes, primarily those of Italian cuisine. But while it adds a unique taste to Italian dishes, oregano has even greater value as a healing herb. It has shown promise as a treatment for bacterial, fungal, and parasitic infections. It also fights inflammation. Carvacrol is the primary active component in oregano oil. A study conducted at Anadolu University in Turkey analyzed the biological activities of carvacrol and concluded that it is antitumor, antibacterial, antiviral, anti-inflammatory, antipain, and a whole host of positive "anti"s![2]

Effective Dosage: To treat bacterial and fungal infections or to guard against damaging inflammation and pain, place a drop of the pure oil under your tongue twice a day.

10. Flaxseed Meal

Why You Might Need This: I make sure to take flaxseed meal (ground flaxseed) every day. It's an exceptional source of mucilage fiber, a gelatinous substance secreted by plants; it soothes the intestinal tract and slows down absorption of glucose in the intestine. Mucilage also helps establish and maintain bowel regularity, prevents bacteria from taking hold in your intestines, and escorts cholesterol, bile acids, and toxins out of your body.

Another of flax's superpowers is its ability to provide essential nutrients such as omega-3 fatty acids and lignans, which are carbohydrates that are thought to fight cancer and diabetes. Nutrition experts say that anyone who is at risk of heart disease, breast cancer, or prostate cancer should take this supplement. In fact, research from Duke University indicates that flaxseed may slow the growth of prostate cancer tumors. A month before 160 men were scheduled to have surgery for prostate cancer, researchers divided them into four groups: Subjects received either 30 grams of ground flaxseed, flaxseed with a low-fat diet, a low-fat diet without flaxseed, or no diet change or supplement intake. The men underwent surgery as planned. Researchers then examined the tumors and found that the cancer cells grew 30 to 40 percent slower in men with flaxseed in their diets.[3]

Effective Dosage: For general health, health care practitioners generally recommend 1 to 2 tablespoons of flaxseed meal once or twice per day. For bowel regularity, take 3 to 5 tablespoons of whole flaxseed with plenty of water over the course of the day. You can stir whole or ground flaxseed into cold cereal, oatmeal, or yogurt or sprinkle it on vegetables or salads.

11. Recovery Drink

Why You Might Need This: After workouts, a sports beverage can help speed recovery by supplying nutrients like amino acids (which the body uses to repair muscle) and carbs (to help restore depleted glycogen stores). Even on nontraining days, these beverages are a convenient way to fit in small, frequent meals. Refueling every few hours prevents overeating. There are hundreds and hundreds of recovery drinks on the market. The product I use is P90X Results and Recovery Formula. It contains whey protein (a fast-replenishing protein), electrolytes (which are lost in sweat), and some sugar (as its main carbohydrate). Why sugar, you say? The first reason is flavor. Recovery drinks have a lot of nutrients, and those all affect the taste. No matter how healthy something is, it's not going to be very helpful if you don't want to drink it! And sugar tastes good. The second reason is nutrient transport. Sugar and other natural sweeteners speed nutrients into your system quickly after a workout, which really helps with recovery.

Effective Dosage: Following your workout, there's a 60-minute window during which you can replenish muscle glycogen and speed recovery two or three times faster than if you wait several hours to eat. Take your recovery drink within that time frame.

Just as your health needs change over time as you enter new stages of life, so do your supplement needs. It's a good idea to periodically review your supplement regimen to see if there are supplements you no longer need, or others you should add to your overall plan. Certain life-changing events, such as having surgery, getting injured, losing a job or changing jobs, getting married or divorced, or losing a loved one, as well as many other situations, can change your nutritional needs.

Take My Supplement Challenge!

If you're still asking yourself whether you really need supplements or whether they're worth the money, here's a simple test. For 1 week, continue working out and eating clean, but do not take any supplements. Answer the 13 questions below at the start and end of that week.

At the start of the following week, add my recommended supplements to your food and workout regimen (women should also add in a calcium supplement). At the end of that second week, take the test again. Compare your numbers, and you'll know if the supplements make a difference.

Answer all questions on a 1-to-10 scale: 1 = never and 10 = always. Be honest!

1. I experience sound, restful sleep most nights of the week.
2. I have plenty of energy throughout the day.
3. I have a healthy and normal appetite with very few cravings.
4. I am happy with my present weight.
5. I'm enthusiastic about my fitness and have plenty of energy during exercise.
6. I'm good at handling stress.
7. I'm satisfied with the state of my libido.
8. My memory, cognition, and mental acuity are good.
9. I have good/full range of motion and am not experiencing joint pain.
10. My muscles are strong and lean and recover quickly after exercise.
11. My heart and lung capacity are strong during cardiovascular exercise.
12. I have normal digestion with no stomach or intestinal issues.
13. I feel that I'm in good mental health, free from sadness, depression, and anxiety.

Choosing the Right Supplements

When it comes to supplements, you definitely get what you pay for, so those supplements you see at the supermart might be cheap, but they are also likely to be loaded with fillers, sugars, or caffeine. What's on the label is not necessarily what is inside the bottle. Remember, the FDA doesn't regulate dietary supplements, so there's no guarantee of a product's safety or efficacy other than the manufacturer's reputation and the ingredients you see listed on the label. Some manufacturers participate in voluntary tests that verify the accuracy of label statements (including content), as well as dissolving rates for tablets. Look for United States Pharmacopoeia (USP) or NSF International seals on the supplements you buy. Also, Consumer Lab reports on the validity of labeling claims (check out ConsumerLab.com for information). Buy supplements from a reliable company, and see how you feel after taking them for a week or so. See if you feel more energetic, less sore, and healthier. Ask your doctor if there have been changes to your blood work at your next physical. If you're seeing positive changes in all of these areas, then you are probably taking the right supplements.

One more point: Before you begin incorporating supplements into your diet, keep in mind that they are *supplementary* to basic health maintenance—that is, they build upon a foundation of proper eating, training, sleep, and rest. Man cannot survive (let alone thrive) on supplements alone!

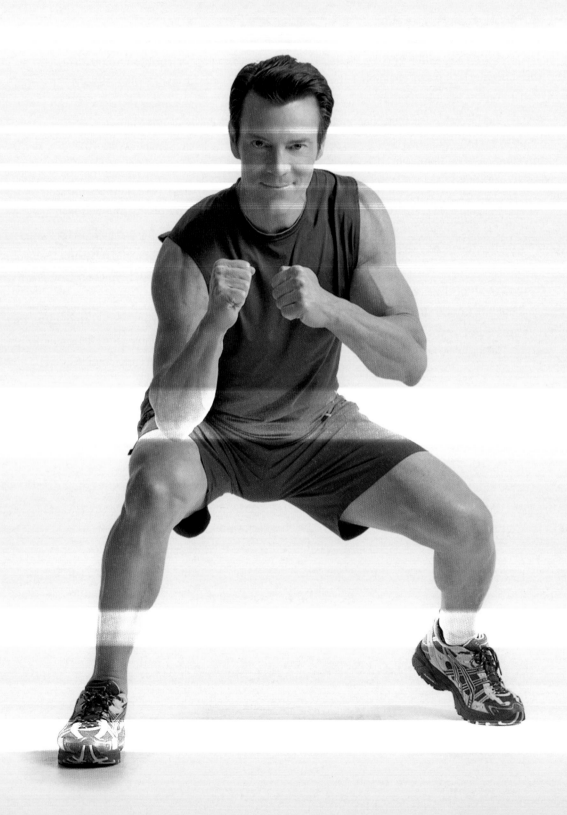

11 Laws of Health and Fitness

You've spent weeks getting in shape, toning up, becoming more flexible, and changing your diet. Finally, you've achieved your dream body—or close to it.

As you continue to follow my program, I want to make sure you keep that body, along with your focus, energy, determination, and enthusiasm. I've found that one of the best ways to get—and keep—the right attitude is to internalize, and live by, a set of guiding principles. You know as well as I do that when laws are broken, there are consequences. The same goes for your personal fitness objectives. Whether it's an expanding waistline, lack of energy, or a dangerously high cholesterol level, there are penalties for eating junk and not working out. My laws, once you start living by them, will help you stay fit for the rest of your life.

Variety Is the Spice of Fitness

Variety means mixing it up and doing something different every day. Sure, you can do just yoga—and you will be more flexible, more patient, and more at peace. But you're going to develop a yoga body with certain limitations. You're not going to be able to run faster or lift a large amount of weight. Or maybe Spinning is your thing. I love Spinning. But if that's all I did, I wouldn't be building upper body strength or flexibility. And by doing the same type of exercise over and over, with no variation in activity, you increase your risk of overuse injuries and ailments such as tendinitis.

Now that you're familiar with my workouts, you can fine-tune them and retrigger muscle growth by making small changes: reversing the order of the exercises, lifting more weight with fewer reps or less weight with more reps, or changing the speed with which you lift and lower weights. Altering your tactics every 6 weeks encourages balanced development; strengthens individual muscles and muscle groups by subjecting them to differing directional stress; and helps prevent dreaded training injuries, plateaus, and boredom.

I hope you've come to understand that the beauty of my program is that it incorporates so many forms of physical activity: resistance to build strength and tone, cardio to create aerobic fitness, and yoga to develop flexibility. You never get bored and you're continually seeing results. So keep your workouts interesting. If you get bored, change it up and shake it up. If variety was the only law you applied to your entire life, you'd have tremendous success.

LAW #2: Consistency

You do need to work out 5 or 6 days a week if you want to experience dramatic results and optimal health. Most of us haven't been raised to think that we need such frequent physical activity in our lives. But to be truly on top of your game, get results in a short period of time, and feel good and be healthy, you must work out most days of the week. Improvement and change occur when you do things often. Stopping and starting all the time will kill any momentum you've built, and you need momentum to succeed.

Think about it like this: You sleep every day. You eat every day. You brush your teeth every day. What happens when you skip a few nights of sleep? If you don't eat? If you don't brush your teeth for a week? There are going to be unpleasant consequences.

Yes, some people will pooh-pooh the notion of daily workouts, and digging in their heels, they just won't do them. That's why I developed the 20-minute workouts for the Beginner's level. Anyone with time constraints can use those workouts. They're not just for Beginners. They're for anyone who would otherwise skip a day of working out because they don't have an hour to spare.

I have several family members who feel they don't have time to exercise, and they're certainly not going to head to the gym for a long workout. However, they can wrap their heads around working out in 20-minute chunks. That's doable for them, and it may be doable for you, too.

Consistency will coalesce into results. If you want to transform your body and your life, stay active most days of the week.

LAW #3: Intensity

People ask me: "Am I overtraining?" "Am I undertraining?"

Here's how to tell: First, be sure to use a heart rate monitor while you're doing cardio. This simple, inexpensive device can tell you whether or not you're in your optimal training zone.

Second, measure your exercise intensity by "rate of exertion." I use a simple 1-to-10 scale. If you're running for your life down an alley while being chased by knife-wielding strangers, that's a 10. If you're lying on the couch, drinking a beer, and watching *American Idol*, that's a 1. Obviously, you don't want to be at a 1 or at a 10. You want to be somewhere between a 6 and an 8. An 8 represents a level of effort that feels like you're working as hard as you can and still hanging in there without stopping or pausing.

On some days, you may only be able to reach a 4. Maybe the previous night you didn't get enough sleep, or you didn't have enough time to properly fuel yourself. Even the temperature in the room or outdoors can affect your intensity. I don't ski as well when the temperature drops to 20 degrees below zero—my whole body feels mummified. But at least I'm on the slopes, despite the conditions, and doing my best.

Intensity is finding your fire and working out as hard as you can, based on where you are today, without sacrificing correct exercise form. Intensity is a moving target, too. It changes from day to day, and there are so many variables outside your control. It's your job to show up, and that's within your control.

LAW #4: Purpose

What is your reason for wanting to stay fit for the rest of your life? Is it vanity? Ego? Weight control? Quality of life? I'll take the latter any day over the first three.

I believe the reason so many people haven't maintained their health and fitness over the long haul is because they're overly focused on vanity, ego, and weight control. I look at weight loss, for example, as a nice aftereffect of fitness, feeling good, and quality of life.

You can have these benefits today. You don't have to wait 30, 60, 90 days or longer like you do with typical diet programs.

After I have an especially crazy day, I ground myself with a workout. A bit of exercise clears my head and immediately makes me feel better. I have a sense of accomplishment. My endorphins are elevated. I feel amazing. After that, I'm ready to face the rat race again.

By contrast, on the days that I don't exercise, I miss out on all of these positive effects. I won't improve my health much. I'll be in a bad mood. My body starts aging again. My muscles will start to atrophy. My organs won't start to manufacture fresh, new cells. My body will start feeling more brittle. The anti-aging process is not reactivated.

Don't let any of those processes take over. Have the right motivation for getting fit. Your reasons why have everything to do with your level of success.

LAW #5: Reality

Be realistic about what you want to achieve. If you're 55 years old and you've never had an athletic day in your life, or you've been overweight since high school, chances are, you're not going to become a rock star or a supermodel in 90 days. You may be able to attain some sylphlike fantasy weight, but what are the odds you'll stay there? You'd probably become frustrated with the deprivation involved, setting the stage for backsliding. Aim for a comfortable weight, though it may be somewhat heavier than you'd hoped, and you'll be more likely to maintain it.

Often, in our desire to get in shape, we set unrealistic goals for ourselves. Our bodies may change, but often they don't stay changed, since we cannot maintain gimmicky or drastic plans. Change must come gradually, and it must come as a result of the realistic incorporation of healthy habits into your daily lifestyle.

Stay realistic about your body type, too. People come in all shapes and sizes, but those shapes and sizes all had definite beginnings—a genetically predetermined body type of ectomorph, endomorph, or mesomorph or, more likely, some combination thereof. You can find out which one you are by taking a good, hard look in the mirror. Are you slender and small-boned, with long arms and a thin neck? You're probably an ectomorph. If you're pear-shaped with shorter arms and legs and big bones, you might be an endomorph. And if you're thick-chested, broad-shouldered, and naturally muscular, you're probably a mesomorph.

The reality is, this is who you are based on the two people (your parents) who conceived you. You are who you are based on their (now your) DNA. Focus on being the best, healthiest version of that.

Reality also means not making excuses for poor progress. I've had people who come up to me and announce, "I did your program for 6 weeks and nothing happened. And I did everything right!" They may believe what they're telling me, but I know that it's not the truth.

Other people say: "I don't have time for this exercise program," "I'm too fat," "I have diabetes," "It hurts my knees," or "I puff and wheeze."

Do you think these responses are excuses or choices?

For a moment, let's compare the terms *excuse* and *choice*. According to the dictionary, an excuse is "a justification of an individual's act or failure to act." And a choice is "the right, power, or opportunity to choose; option."

It's pretty obvious that there's a big difference in the meanings of these two words, yet I think many people confuse them. Every day we make choices that keep us from being who we want to be physically, mentally, and spiritually. These choices are disguised as excuses. Nobody gets away with making lame excuses in this world. Sooner or later (turns out later comes sooner than you thought), your bad behavior will ruin your life.

The first step to changing your excuses to choices is to be honest with yourself. Once you acknowledge that you do have choices, you'll be able to start taking better charge of your life. You have choices. When you realize that, you'll stop making excuses and start making different choices that will help you get to where you want to go.

LAW #6: Play

Sometimes it's important to take your mind off weight, inches, and body fat percentages and focus on active fun. Dance, rock climb, in-line skate, hike, or ride your bike. Outdoor physical activities develop balance, coordination, and stamina—which help accelerate and maintain your health and fitness. Go outside (or inside) and play! Get involved in something that is enjoyable but that also takes you outside of your comfort zone. Set a goal, take a class, sign up for a race—anything that puts the emphasis on what you can *do* and not what you look like. If you shift to a mind-set of playing and having fun, you won't obsess as much about calories, inches, and weight loss.

"Play" doesn't necessarily mean competition. When I was a kid, winning and losing were everything, and that made me miserable. But winning really isn't everything. Statistically, you're probably going to "lose" about half of the time in life—so get comfortable with it.

I enjoy sports like skiing and gymnastics; they aren't competitive in nature, but they help me with balance, stamina, and flexibility. Whatever type of "play" you choose will enhance your ability to become a better athlete. And your athleticism helps you progress faster in your fitness. And best of all, you will be having fun and enjoying yourself the whole time. That synergy is unbeatable.

LAW #7: Plan

Schedule all of your workouts in advance; this creates accountability. Plan an entire month ahead of time. If you schedule it, you'll do it. If you wing it, you won't. It's that simple. When you're accountable, you stay motivated. When you're not accountable to some sort of plan, you can't stay motivated.

I've had a calendar on my desk for 20 years. My schedule is on my laptop, too, so every morning when I log on, it pops up. I know what I'm going to do, when I'm going to do it, and who I'm going to be doing it with. Schedule your workouts as if they are the most important appointment of the day . . . because they are!

On your calendar, write down all of the workouts you're going to do. Every time you complete a workout, mark a big red X over it. At the end of the month, you'd better have 20 to 25 Xs. If not, you haven't been consistent (see Law #2).

Success comes from planning ahead. You can't have a fit, healthy lifestyle if you don't have a long-term plan. Stop winging it, and make sure to schedule all of your workouts in advance.

LAW # 8: Sleep More and Stress Less

You stayed up late last night to finish a project; woke up groggy, only to realize that you'd slept through the alarm clock; skipped breakfast; then almost fell asleep in the middle of an important morning meeting. It's now midafternoon and as you're drinking yet another cup of coffee to stifle yet another yawn, you realize you're just trying to make it through the day to go home and eat pizza.

You're not the only one. Nightly sleep for the average American has dropped from 10 hours (before the invention of the lightbulb) to 6.9 hours, with a third of adults now getting even less than that! In fact, nearly half of all adults admit they sleep less so they can work (or play) more, according to the National Sleep Foundation (NSF). Although most experts agree that the average adult needs 8 hours, most of us have burned our candles at both ends. But how do you get off this "sleep deficit" merry-go-round? It's easy to say "get more sleep," but what if you're simply spending frustrating hours tossing and turning and having trouble finding deep slumber?

First, it's important to be aware that sleep is not a passive activity. Healthy sleep is every bit as valuable to your overall well-being as exercise and good nutrition are. In fact, I'd like to change the name of "sleeping" to "healing." Research shows that a lack of deep sleep (as opposed to irregular or fragmented sleep) undermines the body's ability to fight off disease. Perpetual sleepiness can reduce the quality and quantity of your work by a third, according to the NSF. And if you're sleep-deprived, you're likely to have higher concentrations of sugar in your blood, which could contribute to the development of a prediabetic condition.

If you're experiencing major sleep problems, see your doctor. But for most of us who occasionally have trouble sleeping, there's a simple cure: exercise. Working out regularly has been shown to reduce episodes of insomnia. What's more, it promotes improved sleep quality by producing smoother, more regular transitions between the cycles and phases of sleep. In fact, in a study on sleep patterns of adults ages 50 to 76 who were sedentary and troubled by insomnia, exercise was shown to play a key role. Researchers at Stanford University School of Medicine asked these adults to exercise for 20 to 30 minutes every other day in the afternoon by walking, engaging in low-impact aerobics, and riding a stationary bicycle. The result? Their time required to fall asleep was reduced by half, and total sleep time increased by almost 1 hour.[1]

Another reason to get enough shut-eye: Adequate sleep is associated with more healthful food choices, according to a study conducted at Brigham and Women's Hospital. Researchers studied motor freight workers, who tend to be sleep deprived, and found that when they got enough sleep, they chose better foods.[2] It's not clear exactly why, but it is known that disturbed sleep boosts the stress hormone cortisol to abnormally high levels, and cortisol is responsible for regulating your appetite. Excess cortisol makes you feel hungry, which is why you eat more when you're tired. This also explains why some people eat more when they're stressed.

And speaking of stress, it's a big contributor to sleep deprivation. Over time, chronic stress takes a toll on the body and brain, leading to all kinds of health problems besides insomnia: depression, chronic pain, and cardiovascular disease. For a lot of people, stress can also lead to weight gain.

Stress is an inescapable part of life. Even so, circumstances or people in our lives don't cause stress, nor is it caused by emotions we may experience. Stress comes from our reaction to the stressor. Maybe you've heard the story of the 10 eyewitnesses to a bank robbery: Three robbers storm into the bank, screaming, yelling, and waving guns around. They terrorize the place and steal not only bank funds but also everyone's watches and jewelry. Each eyewitness experienced the same event but had very different reactions to it. Some were traumatized, while others amused friends at cocktail parties with the story. The moral of the story is this: You choose how you respond to stressful events. And this response profoundly affects your stress level, for good and bad.

You can choose to panic and freak out all you want, but time will still pass and life will still happen. So why not choose patience or curiosity? Patience is a virtue, and who wouldn't want to be virtuous in a stressful situation? To be curious means asking the right questions to help find solutions to the stressful situation. When does fear, worry, or anxiety ever help solve a problem? Being stressed-out drains your energy. Allowing stress to overtake you means that you're having a tough time coping with the realities of life. Don't let stress be your scapegoat. Stand up, take a deep breath, and see if you can deal with reality under pressure. And if life really feels overwhelming and you need some help managing your stress, don't be afraid to ask for it.

LAW #9: Love It!

Your workouts require commitment, determination, planning, consistency, and intensity. If you don't like what you're doing, then there's no way on earth you'll succeed. Enthusiasm is a huge piece of the puzzle. Get creative and stay curious. If you enjoy doing my program exclusively and it works for you, then keep doing it until it doesn't. If you get partway through and it's not your cup of tea, then stop and do something else. Something has to bring you back day after day, week after week. Love it or leave it.

I don't know about you, but if I don't like or love something, then I don't do it. Period. On the other hand, I'm extremely motivated when it comes to doing the things I love. Folks always ask me what I think are the best ways to get into shape: "Are your workouts really the best for me?" "What do you think about Spinning?" "I hear that kayaking is the fastest growing sport in America; will that get me in shape?" "If I run more, will that help me burn off extra fat?" The truth is, they're all great ways to lose weight, get in shape, and live a healthy lifestyle. If any of these things feel like work *to* you, then they won't work *for* you. Especially in the long haul. People fail to finish fitness programs because they don't enjoy what they're doing.

The formula for figuring out what you love is right in this book. It also involves staying creative and curious. Both involve finding ways to modify, integrate, and alter your workouts so that you can incorporate the things you love into your daily routines. I'm at the point in my fitness journey where I'm not exactly sure what my workout is going to look like 10 minutes before I start it. I often develop my workouts on the fly. This approach allows me to be creative as I make my way through it. I do this when I ski and rock climb, so why not with my workouts?

If you stay curious, try new things, abandon the exercises you dislike, and keep the ones you love, then you'll discover a fitness philosophy that you'll stick with for a lifetime.

LAW #10: Flexibility

Throughout this book, I've preached the importance of flexibility, so I'm going to keep my comments short here. The importance of staying flexible applies to every age group. In younger, growing athletes, for example, it's important to stretch to maintain the flexibility of the joint and prevent injuries. Young athletes can have tight hamstrings and tight heel cords, so it's good to be mobilized before they go out and compete.

Many people assume that increasing muscle weakness and stiffness is an inevitable part of aging. But increasingly, research suggests that much of the decline attributed to aging actually comes from disuse. Flexibility is the key component to becoming less vulnerable and more durable, no matter what your age.

LAW #11: Eat Well

Healthy, nutritious food provides the energy you need to get through a hectic day and a high-energy workout. Eating high-quality foods combined with proper supplementation greatly reduces your risk of illness and disease. Nutritious foods and the right supplements can assist in lowering fat stores, losing weight, increasing energy, recovering from workouts, and maintaining healthy bones, muscles, and joints. Supplementation and eating well also promote psychological health.

Nick's story is a testament to what happens when you fuel yourself properly. It's so powerful that I'll let him tell it in his own words.

I have never been one to really struggle with weight, but after a messy breakup and a short bout of depression, I really spiraled out of control. I was eating unhealthy foods and just wasn't taking care of my body. I was sluggish and had no energy. I got to the point where my self-confidence was at an all-time low and my weight at an all-time high. Other than going to work, I didn't want to leave my house, and any social life I had came to a screeching halt.

A few of my friends were talking about your exercise and nutrition programs. I looked into them. I liked what I saw. I knew if I was going to do it, I would have to fully commit to making a life change, so I did—I cut out all junk food, fast food, and sodas. This was the best move I have ever made. Now I can't even believe I ever put some of those foods in my body.

Overall, I have lost 28 pounds since starting the program last fall. I still have a few more months before I think I will reach my weight-loss goal (another 15 pounds), but I now know I will get there. Thanks, man, for giving me my life back.

It didn't take long for Nick to experience dramatic changes. After just a couple of months of treating his body well, his blood sugar and cholesterol dropped, along with those extra pounds. Now he feels better than he has in years, and he credits the power of food with helping him heal.

As I close this book, I want to thank you for choosing perseverance over laziness, discipline over impatience, self-reliance over self-pity, and hard work over quick fixes. Shortcuts, pills and potions, and weight-loss-only diet programs have fooled people in the past but are now becoming ancient relics. I realize the road to lasting health and fitness is often bumpy and the journey is long, but the results of commitment and dedication are life-altering. Don't ease up. When life is hardest, you must narrow your focus and keep going.

My sincerest hope is that I have made a difference in your life. More and more people are waking up to the reality that a happy, healthy life must be fueled by whole foods and plenty of exercise—and you're one of those people. You've started a lifestyle that is going to last the rest of your life. Stay focused on keeping a lean, healthy, energized body—and on the pleasure of looking and feeling your absolute best. You've come this far, and there are no limits to where you can go from here.

Recipes

Cooking has never been my forte. Eating, on the other hand—well, that's a different story. Although boiling water is about as creative as I get in the kitchen, I recognize the importance of a home-cooked meal, one that's loaded with complex carbs, protein, and healthy fats. The bottom line is that when you eat out, you really don't know what you're getting, but when you cook at home, you have control over every single ingredient that goes into your food. I challenge you to find your love for cooking and learn to enjoy being in the kitchen.

Being healthy is a lifestyle, a way of being, and if you can't cook your own food to stay on track, then you will easily get off track and eat in a rush. It's important to make a plan for what you will eat each week, reconnect with your food, and get the other members of your household involved. If you have kids, teach them how to eat now so that they can make healthy choices throughout their lives. Let them help you in the kitchen and educate them on the importance of eating fruits, vegetables, and whole grains. Family support will also help you stay on track and meet your goals.

Beverages and Snacks

Tony's Power Protein Smoothie

This delightful and nutrient-packed smoothie is my favorite postworkout drink for recovery, muscle building, and fat burning.

½ cup almond milk

½ cup coconut water

1 scoop protein powder

1 scoop greens powder

1 scoop reds powder

½ cup frozen berries

½ banana

20 raw cashews or 2 teaspoons almond butter

Ice (optional)

Combine all ingredients in a blender and process until smooth.

Makes 1 large serving

Tropical Blaster

Coconut, mango, pineapple. You'll feel like you're in the tropics doing the hula, Horton style, when you sip this nutrient-dense smoothie!

½ cup almond milk

½ cup coconut water

½ banana

¼ cup shredded coconut, unsweetened

½ cup frozen pineapple or mango

2 teaspoons coconut oil

Dash of cinnamon

Combine all ingredients in a blender and process until smooth.

Makes 1 large serving

Get Up and Go Granola

Most commercial granolas are full of fat and added sugar. Not this one. You'll love it.

3 cups rolled oats (not instant)

I cup oat flour or spelt flour

I cup walnuts, chopped, or any other nut

½ cup flaxseed

½ teaspoon sea salt

½ teaspoon cinnamon

½ teaspoon cardamom

¾ cup grapeseed oil

¾ cup maple syrup or agave nectar

I teaspoon vanilla or almond extract, alcohol-free if available

Preheat the oven to 350°F and line a baking sheet with parchment paper.

In a larg mixing bowl, combine the oats, flour, nuts, flaxseed, salt, cinnamon, and cardamom. Mix well.

In a small bowl, combine the oil, syrup or agave nectar, and extract. Whisk together until well combined. Pour the oil mixture over the oats mixture and stir to combine.

Spread the granola evenly on the baking sheet. Bake for about 30 minutes, or until golden brown. Remove it from the oven and let it sit for 5 minutes to crisp up, and then break it into chunks.

Makes 4 to 6 servings

My Sticky Bar

This is a fast snack—fast to make and fast to eat.

½ banana

½ cup Get Up and Go Granola (above)

I heaping tablespoon crunchy almond butter

Use a fork to mash up the banana, then mix it with the granola and almond butter. Roll the mixture into a bar. Freeze. When you're ready to eat, heat the sticky bar in the microwave on high for 20 seconds. You can double or triple this recipe.

Makes I bar

Melissa's "Cheesy" Popcorn

Popcorn is everyone's favorite snack—it's filling, high in fiber, and just plain fun to eat.

   1 tablespoon extra virgin coconut oil

   ½ cup organic corn kernels (it's best to buy these in bulk)

   Sea salt and ground black pepper

   Nutritional yeast flakes

In a large pot with a fitted lid, heat the coconut oil over medium heat until melted. Add the popcorn kernels and place the lid on the pot. Wait until the first kernel pops and then the lower heat slightly. The popcorn will continue to pop. (You do not need to shake the pot, but you can.) Cook until you hear the popping slow.

Remove the pot from the heat and season the corn with salt, pepper, and nutritional yeast flakes to taste for a "cheesy" flavor. Mix well or shake in a bag.

Makes 4 servings

Spicy Edamame Dip

Protein-packed edamame beans with cayenne and lime make this dip a favorite.

   1 package (16-ounces) frozen shelled edamame

   5 tablespoons extra virgin olive oil

   4 large garlic cloves, chopped

   ½ teaspoon ground coriander

   ½ teaspoon ground cumin

   1¼ teaspoons sea salt

   ¼ teaspoon cayenne pepper

   ¼ cup fresh lime juice

   ¼ cup fresh chopped cilantro (optional)

Cook the edamame in boiling water according to the package directions. Drain, reserving ⅓ cup of the cooking water, and set aside. Heat 1 tablespoon of the oil in a skillet over medium heat. Sauté the garlic, coriander, and cumin in the skillet until the garlic is soft and the spices are fragrant. Scrape the garlic mixture out of the pan and into the bowl of a food processor.

Add the salt and cayenne pepper to the food processor. Puree until smooth. Add the lime juice and the remaining 4 tablespoons of oil and puree to combine, scraping the sides of the bowl frequently. Keep the motor running and slowly pour in the reserved water until you get a smooth consistency. You may not need to use all of the water, depending on the consistency you prefer.

Add the fresh cilantro, if using, and serve with pita crisps, vegetables, or sprouted rice crackers.

Makes approximately 2½ cups

Garlicky Karma Hummus

Garlicky and good! This is my favorite spread for dipping fresh veggies or adding to wraps.

I can (14 ounces) chickpeas, drained and rinsed

½ teaspoon salt

¼ teaspoon ground black pepper

I tiny pinch cayenne pepper

3 tablespoons water

3 tablespoons extra virgin olive oil

4 cloves garlic, chopped

I teaspoon ground cumin

3 tablespoons freshly squeezed lemon juice

¼ cup unroasted sesame tahini

Put the chickpeas, salt, black pepper, cayenne pepper, and water in a blender or food processor.

Heat the oil in a skillet over medium heat, and sauté the garlic in the oil until it's lightly roasted. Add the cumin to the oil and stir to combine. Pour the oil mixture into the blender or food processor with the beans. Add the lemon juice and pulse the mixture until smooth, scraping the sides of the bowl. Add a little extra lemon juice or olive oil if the mixture is too thick. Add the tahini and mix until well blended. Adjust seasonings to taste.

Makes approximately 2½ cups

Soups and Salads

Kitchen Sink Veggie Soup

Chock-full of vegetables, this soup is a bowlful of nutrition. You can also add some brown rice or barley for extra fiber and complex carbs.

 2 tablespoons extra virgin olive oil

 I red onion, finely chopped

 2 shallots, chopped

 I leek, thinly sliced

 3 cloves garlic, chopped

 3 celery stalks, chopped into small pieces

 2 teaspoons ground cumin

 4 carrots, peeled and chopped

 I can (I5 ounces) fire-roasted diced tomatoes

 Combination of any seasonal fresh vegetables you want: zucchini; Red Bliss potatoes, cut into cubes; broccoli, cut into small florets; cabbage, thinly chopped; sweet potatoes, cut into small cubes; cauliflower, cut into small pieces; Brussels sprouts, ends trimmed off and cut into quarters

 Any fresh herbs you want: dill, thyme, marjoram

 4–6 cups low-sodium vegetable broth

 Sea salt and ground black pepper

In a large soup pot over medium heat, warm the oil. Sauté the onion, shallots, leek, garlic, and celery until soft. Add the cumin and stir to incorporate and release the flavor. Add the carrots and tomatoes, as well as any additional vegetables and herbs you are using. Add 4 to 6 cups of vegetable broth, depending on the amount of vegetables you are using. (Add enough to just cover the vegetables, as they will cook down.) Turn up the heat and bring the soup to a boil. Cover and reduce the heat. Simmer until the veggies are tender, 20 to 30 minutes. Season with salt and pepper to taste. Top with fresh chopped dill or another fresh herb.

For a heartier soup, add ½ cup cooked brown rice or other grain to the bowl when serving.

Makes 6 to 8 Servings

Melissa's Roasted Butternut Squash Soup

I love this creamy, sweet, and satisfying soup served with a side salad.

I large butternut squash, roasted (this can be done day before; see below)

2 tablespoons extra virgin olive oil

I large shallot, finely diced

½ sweet onion, diced

2 stalks celery, diced

5 carrots, peeled and chopped

I teaspoon cumin powder

I large garnet yam, peeled and cubed

4 cups vegetable broth

I can (15 ounces) coconut milk

Dash of cinnamon and/or nutmeg or garam masala (Indian spice blend)

Dash of cloves

Sea salt and ground black pepper

I tablespoon maple syrup (optional)

Pumpkin seeds, toasted pecans or walnuts, fresh herbs, or sliced pears

To prepare the squash: Heat the oven to 350°F. Cut the squash in half lengthwise. Line a baking dish or cookie sheet with parchment paper and coat it with cooking spray. Place the squash cut side down on the parchment and poke holes in the squash with a sharp knife or fork, then spray the squash with cooking spray. Bake for about 45 minutes, or until the squash can be easily pierced with a fork. Take it out of the oven and let it cool.

To prepare the soup: In a large pot over medium heat, heat the oil. Add the shallot, onion, and celery and sauté for about 5 minutes, or until they're soft and translucent. Add the carrots and cook for about 3 minutes longer. Add the cumin and stir to release the flavor. Add the yam and broth. Cover the pot and bring the soup to a boil. Turn down the heat and simmer until the vegetables are tender, about 20 minutes.

Meanwhile, remove and discard the seeds from the squash. Scoop out the flesh and put it into a bowl. Discard the skin. Add the squash to the pot and cook for a couple of minutes. Add the coconut milk and stir well to combine. Reduce the heat to low, and do not bring the soup to a boil once you add the coconut milk, as the milk will curdle.

In batches, ladle the mixture into a blender and puree until very smooth, or use a hand blender. Pour the pureed soup back into the pot. Add the cinnamon, nutmeg, or garam masala. Add the cloves, salt and pepper to taste, and syrup (if using). The soup will be very thick. If you want a thinner soup, add a little water.

To serve, top the soup with pumpkin seeds, toasted pecans or walnuts, fresh herbs, or sliced pears.

Makes 6 to 8 servings

Lentil Soup

Lentils are packed with fiber and protein, making this hearty and filling soup a favorite post-workout meal.

I tablespoon extra virgin olive oil or coconut oil

I large sweet onion, chopped

4 cloves garlic, minced

I large shallot, diced

3 stalks celery, finely chopped

3 carrots, peeled and diced

2 teaspoons dried tarragon

I teaspoon dried thyme

I teaspoon paprika

5 plum tomatoes, diced, or I can (I5 ounces) fire-roasted diced tomatoes

6 cups low-sodium vegetable stock or broth

2 cups French lentils

2 bay leaves

I teaspoon sea salt

Ground black pepper

In a large soup pot over medium heat, heat the oil. Add the onion, garlic, and shallot. Sauté for about 10 minutes, or until the onion and shallot are a little brown. Add the celery, carrots, tarragon, thyme, and paprika. Add the tomatoes and a splash of water. Stir to combine. Cover and cook for about 5 minutes.

Add the stock or broth, lentils, bay leaves, salt, and pepper to taste. Turn up the heat and bring the soup to a boil. Once it's boiling, cover the pot with a lid, turn down the heat to a simmer, and cook covered for about 45 minutes, or until the lentils are tender.

Makes 6 to 8 servings

White Bean Soup

A friend of mine whipped this up for me one day. It is so delicious that I eat it almost every week.

2 tablespoons olive oil

4 cloves garlic, diced

2 shallots, diced

2 cups low-sodium chicken or vegetable broth

¼ teaspoon parsley

¼ teaspoon sage

¼ teaspoon rosemary

¼ teaspoon thyme

½ teaspoon sea salt

2 cans (15 ounces each) white kidney beans, rinsed and drained

2 cans (15 ounces each) white navy beans, rinsed and drained

1½ cups organic almond milk

Salt and ground black pepper

Chives

In a 3-quart stockpot over medium heat, heat the oil. Sauté the garlic and shallots in the oil until translucent. Add the broth, parsley, sage, rosemary, thyme, salt, 1 can of the kidney beans, and 1 can of the navy beans. Simmer for 15 minutes, turn off the heat, and let the mixture cool for 15 minutes. After it has cooled, put it in a blender or food processor and puree. Add the almond milk and puree until the mixture is smooth. Return the pureed mixture to the stockpot and add the remaining kidney and navy beans. Return to a rolling boil, then reduce the heat and simmer for an additional 20 minutes. Add salt and pepper to taste before serving. Garnish with the chives and serve hot.

Makes 6 to 8 servings

Warm Artichoke and Chickpea Salad

Chickpeas, sun-dried tomatoes, and roasted red peppers all make this protein-filled salad a tasty addition to any meal! I also love to snack on this salad during the day.

I tablespoon extra virgin olive oil

I large shallot, diced

3 cloves garlic, minced

I tablespoon minced fresh rosemary or thyme

I can (15 ounces) artichoke hearts in water, drained and rinsed

2 cans (15 ounces each) chickpeas, drained and rinsed

¼ cup sun-dried tomatoes, packed in oil and julienned

¼ cup chopped roasted red bell peppers

I tablespoon freshly squeezed lemon juice

Sea salt and ground black pepper

In a skillet over medium heat, heat the oil. Sauté the shallot until translucent. Add the garlic and sauté 3 minutes longer. Add the rosemary and artichoke hearts to the skillet and stir frequently, letting the artichoke hearts get slightly browned. In the meantime, add the chickpeas, sundried tomatoes, and roasted peppers to a large bowl. Pour in the shallot and artichoke mixture and mix well to combine. Sprinkle on the fresh lemon juice and season with salt and pepper to taste.

Raw Spinach Salad with Fennel

This crunchy and satisfying salad is health in a bowl!

Dressing

I shallot, diced

I tablespoon Dijon mustard

I tablespoon sweet white miso

¼ cup rice wine vinegar

I teaspoon maple syrup or agave
   nectar

3 tablespoons extra virgin olive oil

Salad

1 or 2 bags (5 ounces each) spinach

2 tablespoons extra virgin olive oil

Dash of sea salt

½ cup cherry tomatoes, quartered or halved

I bulb fennel, thinly sliced

¼ cup pine nuts

¼ cup dried cranberries (optional)

To make the dressing: Puree the shallot, mustard, miso, vinegar, syrup or agave nectar, and oil in a blender or combine them in a bottle and shake well to mix.

To make the salad: Wash the spinach and use a salad spinner to spin it dry. Place it in a large bowl, drizzle with the oil, and sprinkle with the salt. Add the tomatoes, fennel, and pine nuts and toss with the dressing. Sprinkle with the cranberries, if using.

Makes 2 to 4 servings

Brussels Sprouts Salad with Cranberries and Almonds

The sweetness of the antioxidant-packed cranberries and the crunchiness of the almonds make this salad a delicious and nutritious accompaniment to any meal.

I pound Brussels sprouts, ends cut off and then sliced

½ cup almonds, smoked or roasted

½ cup dried cranberries

I large shallot, diced

Goat milk feta (optional)

Lemon Vinaigrette (see the recipe below)

Sea salt and ground black pepper

Blanch the Brussels sprouts in boiling water for 3 minutes. Drain and set them aside to cool. Once they're cool, place them in a bowl and add the almonds, cranberries, shallot, and cheese (if using). Toss with the vinaigrette. Season with salt and pepper to taste.

Makes 2 to 4 servings

Lemon Vinaigrette

Juice of I lemon

¼ cup olive oil

½ cup seasoned rice wine vinegar

I tablespoon Dijon mustard

I shallot, minced finely (optional)

Puree the lemon juice, oil, vinegar, mustard, and shallot in a blender, or combine them in a bottle and shake well to mix.

Makes approximately I cup

Quinoa Black Bean Salad with Dried Apricots

I love the protein that quinoa packs, and this salad's blend of lime, mint, and apricot leaves a delightful and refreshing taste dancing on your tongue.

Dressing

2 tablespoons rice wine vinegar

2 tablespoons freshly squeezed lime juice

¼ cup apricot nectar

I jalapeño pepper, seeded and diced (wear plastic gloves when handling)

¼ cup extra virgin olive oil or flax oil

¼ teaspoon sea salt

Salad

½ cup chopped dried apricots or 3 fresh apricots, pitted and chopped

I small red bell pepper, seeded and diced

I small red onion, diced

I cup chopped scallions

I cup fresh cilantro

¼ cup toasted pumpkin seeds

2 cups cooked quinoa, cooled

I can (15 ounces) black beans, rinsed and drained

To make the dressing: Puree the vinegar, lime juice, apricot nectar, jalapeño, oil, and salt in a blender, or combine them in a bottle and shake well to mix.

To make the salad: In a mixing bowl, combine the apricots, bell pepper, onion, scallions, cilantro, and pumpkin seeds. Toss to combine.

Add the quinoa to the mixing bowl and toss together until everything is well combined. Fold in the black beans. Add the dressing to taste, stir, and let the salad sit for 10 minutes so the flavors incorporate. This salad is good served chilled, too.

Makes 6 servings

Fresh Pesto, Tomato, and Zucchini Pasta

Here's a flavorful way to get in your veggies and eat your pasta, too!

I pound brown rice fusilli pasta

I tablespoon extra virgin olive oil

3 cloves garlic, minced

I red onion, diced

I cup chopped mushrooms

2 zucchini, cut into quarters and diced

I teaspoon oregano

I teaspoon basil

4 Roma tomatoes, diced

I can (15 ounces) fire-roasted diced tomatoes

¼ cup pesto (see the recipe below)

Cook the pasta according to the package directions. In a skillet, heat the oil over medium heat. Add the garlic and onion. Cook until they're translucent. Add the mushrooms, zucchini, oregano, and basil and cook until slightly brown. Add the Roma tomatoes and canned tomatoes and cover for about 5 minutes so that the tomatoes cook down. Add the pesto and stir to mix.

Serve immediately over the pasta.

Makes 4 servings

Pesto

2 large bunches basil, stems removed (about 3 cups loosely packed leaves)

¼ cup pine nuts

2 or 3 cloves garlic

Juice of ½ lemon

3 tablespoons extra virgin olive oil

Sea salt and ground black pepper

In a food processor, combine the basil, pine nuts, and garlic. Blend until the ingredients begin to form a paste. Scrape the sides of the bowl as necessary. Add the lemon juice and blend. While the motor is running, drizzle in the oil and salt and pepper to taste. Process until smooth and creamy. Add additional oil if necessary.

Makes ½ cup

Side Dishes

Lemon Garlic Green Beans

Green beans at their finest—this is my favorite veggie side dish with any meal.

  2 tablespoons extra virgin olive oil

  5 cloves garlic, finely minced

  1 pound fresh green beans, ends trimmed (about 4 cups)

  Juice of 1 lemon

  Sea salt and ground black pepper

In a skillet that has a lid, heat the oil over medium heat. Add the garlic and sauté for 3 minutes. Add the green beans and cover for 5 to 8 minutes to "steam." Remove the lid and stir. The green beans should be bright green and crisp. Pour on the lemon juice and stir to combine. Add salt and pepper to taste. Remove from the heat and serve immediately.

Makes 4 servings

Oven-Baked Yam Chili "Fries"

These "fries" are actually baked and thus free of the saturated fat that normal fries contain. I love to eat these alongside my Karma Chow Veggie Burgers (see the recipe on page 278), dipped in a bit of fruit-sweetened ketchup.

  2 large garnet yams, peeled and cut into $\frac{1}{4}$" thick "fries"

  Extra virgin olive oil

  2 teaspoons chili powder blend

  Sea salt

Preheat the oven to 400°F. Line a baking sheet with parchment paper.

Place the yams in a large bowl and drizzle with just enough oil to coat. Season with the chili powder and sea salt to taste. Using your hands, toss the yams to evenly coat them with the seasoning. Spread the fries in a single layer on the baking sheet. Bake in the oven for about 20 minutes, turning occasionally, until they're browned and tender. Let them cool for 5 minutes before serving.

Makes 2 servings

Main Dishes

Black Bean Yam Chili

Loaded with my favorite nutrient-packed food, yams, this chili is a blend of smoky, sweet, and spicy. It's so hearty you can eat it as a meal by itself. Serve it alongside a large green or spinach salad with lots of fresh vegetables!

- 2 tablespoons olive oil or coconut oil
- 4 cloves garlic, minced
- I medium red onion, diced
- I red bell pepper, seeded and diced
- 2 teaspoons sea salt
- I tablespoon cumin
- 2 tablespoons chili powder
- I large garnet yam, cut into ½" cubes
- Zest and juice of I lime
- I can (28 ounces) fire-roasted crushed organic tomatoes (Muir Glen brand is best)
- I cup water or vegetable stock
- 3 cans (14 ounces each) black beans, drained and rinsed (or 4 cups freshly cooked)
- I teaspoon cocoa powder
- I cup chopped cilantro for garnish (optional)

In a large pot over medium heat, heat the oil. Sauté the garlic, onion, pepper, and salt until the veggies are soft, 4 to 5 minutes. Add the cumin and chili powder and stir to combine. Cook for another minute. Add the yam and lime zest and cook for about 10 minutes more, stirring occasionally. Add the tomatoes, water or vegetable stock, beans, lime juice, and cocoa powder. Bring to a simmer, cover, and cook for 10 minutes, or until the yams are soft.

Top with chopped cilantro (if using) and a squeeze of lime, if desired. Serve over brown rice or with gluten-free cornbread.

Makes 6 servings

Variation:
Add I pound of lean ground turkey or chicken to make a heartier chili with extra protein.

Yam Tempeh Stew

If you're like me, this dish will remind you of the beef stew you loved as a kid. This stew tastes just like my grandmother's recipe—you'll never miss the beef!

2 tablespoons extra virgin olive oil

2 cups chopped red onion

I cup sliced celery with leaves

2 cups sliced carrots

I pound tempeh, cubed

I teaspoon dried oregano

4 cups garnet yams, peeled and cubed (about 2 medium yams)

1½ cups parsnips, peeled and cubed

4 cups vegetable stock or low-sodium broth

I bay leaf

I can (28 ounces) fire-roasted whole tomatoes in juice

¾ cup hulled barley, rinsed

I tablespoon vegan Worcestershire sauce (if available)

1½ cups frozen peas

In a stockpot over medium heat, heat the oil. Add the onion, celery, and carrots, and sauté until the onion is translucent. Add the tempeh and oregano and sauté for a few minutes longer, stirring occasionally. Add the yams and parsnips and stir to combine. Cook for 3 minutes, and then add the stock or broth, bay leaf, tomatoes, and barley. Bring to a boil, then cover the pot, lower the heat, and simmer until all the vegetables and the barley are tender, about 20 minutes. Add the Worcestershire sauce and simmer for 10 more minutes. Add the peas last and stir to combine. Cook for 2 more minutes. Serve immediately.

Makes 8 to 10 servings

Variation:

For a meatier stew, you can replace the tempeh with I pound of lean ground white turkey meat.

Karma Chow Veggie Burgers

These hearty veggie burgers will fill you up without all of the saturated fat of red meat. I nosh on these served over a bed of leafy greens.

I red bell pepper, seeded and cut into chunks

½ red onion, cut into chunks

4 tablespoons fresh cilantro

I cup baby spinach

Sea salt and ground black pepper

I teaspoon chili powder blend

2 tablespoons tomato paste

I can (15 ounces) chickpeas, drained and rinsed, or 1½ cups cooked

I cup cooked brown rice

2 cups bread crumbs, whole wheat or gluten-free

1–2 tablespoons extra virgin oil

In a food processor, pulse the bell pepper, onion, cilantro, and spinach until well combined. Transfer the mixture to a large bowl and stir in salt and black pepper to taste, chili powder, and tomato paste. In the same food processor cup, pulse the chickpeas and rice until combined. Add this to the vegetable mixture. Add the bread crumbs and mix well, using your hands to combine.

Form the mixture into patties. Heat them on a grill or in a skillet with the oil until golden brown. Serve immediately with all the fixings on a sprouted-grain bun or bed of lettuce.

Makes 8 patties

Supreme Vegetarian Burrito

This burrito is a staple in my everyday diet. I sometimes eat two a day. Loaded with complex carbs, protein, and healthy fat, it's the perfect meal along with a side salad.

- I cup brown rice
- 2 tablespoons extra virgin olive oil
- I red bell pepper, seeded and sliced into thin strips
- I green or yellow bell pepper, seeded and sliced into thin strips
- I red onion, thinly sliced
- 2 teaspoons ground cumin
- 2 tablespoons chili powder blend
- ½ teaspoon sea salt
- Ground black pepper
- I can (15 ounces) fire-roasted diced tomatoes
- I can (15 ounces) organic black beans, drained and rinsed
- I package sprouted or whole wheat tortillas

Extras (optional)

- Cheese (preferably nondairy)
- Avocado
- Salsa
- Tempeh bacon

Rinse the brown rice and prepare it according to the package directions.

While the rice is cooking, heat I tablespoon of the oil in a large skillet. Add the bell peppers and onion and sauté until soft, 3 to 5 minutes. Add the cumin, chili powder, salt, and black pepper to taste, and continue cooking for 2 more minutes, stirring to incorporate all the spices with the peppers and onion. Add the tomatoes and stir to mix. Lower the heat and cover, cooking for about 5 minutes, until the peppers are really soft. Remove from the heat. Add the beans to the skillet and stir to incorporate.

To assemble: Heat a tortilla over a low open flame on the stove. Place the tortilla on a flat surface. Spread a very small amount of grated cheese (if using) over the entire tortilla. Add I scoop of the filling to the bottom third of the tortilla. Top with I scoop of the rice. Add avocado, salsa, or tempeh bacon (if using) and roll up the tortilla.

Makes 6 to 8 burritos

Gingery Vegetable Stir-Fry

This nutritious dish contains a rainbow of fresh vegetables and packs a punch of ginger flavor.

Sauce

1 tablespoon minced garlic

2 teaspoons grated fresh ginger

¼ cup mellow white miso

2 teaspoons arrowroot powder

2 tablespoons maple syrup

3 tablespoons low-sodium tamari

2 tablespoons toasted sesame oil

Pinch of red-pepper flakes

½ cup water

Stir-Fry

2 tablespoons coconut oil

3 cloves garlic, minced

1 yellow onion, diced

1 red bell pepper, seeded and diced

1 yellow bell pepper, seeded and diced

1 bunch asparagus, chopped into 1″ pieces

½ cup chopped bok choy

1½ cups chopped broccoli

½ cup chopped carrots

½ cup mushrooms, stemmed and chopped

1 cup shredded cabbage (optional)

1 cup brown rice or quinoa, cooked

3 scallions, chopped

Sesame seeds (optional)

To make the sauce: Place the garlic, ginger, miso, arrowroot, syrup, tamari, oil, pepper flakes, and water in a blender. Blend until smooth.

To make the stir-fry: In a large wok or sauté pan, heat the oil over medium-high heat. Add the garlic and onion and sauté until translucent, about 5 minutes. Add the peppers, asparagus, bok choy, broccoli, carrots, mushrooms, and cabbage. Stir to combine. Cover and let the veggies steam for about 5 minutes. If they start to stick, add a small amount of water.

Add the sauce to the wok and continue to stir-fry for a few more minutes to incorporate the flavors. Serve over the rice or quinoa and garnish with the scallions. Sprinkle with the sesame seeds (if using) before serving.

Makes 4 to 6 servings

Divine Rice Wrap

Here's a recipe that's simple and easy to throw together with whatever vegetables you have hanging around in the fridge. It's loaded with nutrition, fiber, and flavor.

I brown rice wrap tortilla, gluten-free

3 tablespoons Garlicky Karma Hummus (see the recipe on page 266)

Cucumber

Tomato

Red onion

Bell pepper

Lettuce of choice—spinach, arugula, baby greens, etc.

Balsamic vinegar

Sea salt and ground black pepper

Heat the wrap over an open flame. Slather with the hummus and fill with veggies. Drizzle on some balsamic vinegar and sprinkle with salt and pepper. Roll up the wrap and enjoy.

Makes I wrap

Baked Apricot-Glazed Chicken Breasts

This simple chicken dish is light, sweet, and easy to make. It will become your go-to chicken recipe.

4 boneless, skinless breasts (5 ounces each)

Salt and ground black pepper

I tablespoon extra virgin olive oil

I large shallot, chopped

2 tablespoons apple cider vinegar

I tablespoon soy sauce

½ cup chicken or vegetable stock

½ cup orange juice, freshly squeezed

I cup apricot all-fruit preserves (no sugar added)

Preheat the oven to 350°F. Rinse the chicken and pat dry. Season with salt and pepper to taste.

In a small saucepan, heat the oil and sauté the shallot until translucent. Add the remaining ingredients and simmer until the preserves are melted. Place the chicken in a baking dish and pour the preserves over the chicken. Bake for 20 minutes, basting every so often with the glaze.

Makes 4 servings

Broiled Soy Maple Salmon

This sweet, delicious dish is loaded with heart-healthy omega-3 fats.

¼ cup low-sodium soy sauce or tamari

2 tablespoons pure maple syrup

2 tablespoons mirin (Japanese rice wine)

⅛ teaspoon crushed red-pepper flakes

2 tablespoons toasted sesame oil

2 cloves garlic, minced

3 scallions, thinly sliced

I tablespoon fresh lime juice

I teaspoon arrowroot powder

I tablespoon freshly grated ginger

4 salmon fillets (6 ounces each), about ¾" thick

Preheat the broiler to high. In a bowl, whisk together all wet ingredients and spices.

Place the salmon in a casserole dish and top with the sauce. Cover and marinate for at least 20 minutes.

Place the salmon on a broiler pan lined with nonstick foil. Pour the remaining sauce into a saucepan and heat to thicken, stirring constantly. Broil the salmon for about 10 minutes, or until flaky. Top with any additional sauce.

Makes 4 servings

Desserts

Apple-Pear Crisp

Here's a mouthwatering dessert that is actually healthy! I love to eat this hearty fruit dessert in the fall.

Filling

8–10 apples and pears (Granny Smith apples and Bosc pears are a
    good combination)

¼ cup agave nectar or maple syrup

1 teaspoon almond extract

2 teaspoons grated fresh ginger

Zest of 1 orange (optional)

½ cup pure apple cider or juice

1 tablespoon arrowroot powder

Topping

2 cups rolled oats

1 cup oat or almond flour

1 cup toasted sliced almonds

¼ teaspoon sea salt

½ cup agave nectar or brown rice syrup

⅓ cup grapeseed, coconut, or walnut oil

1 teaspoon almond extract

Preheat the oven to 250°F.

To make the filling: Peel, core, and slice the apples and pears. Place the fruit in a large casserole dish. In a medium bowl, combine the agave nectar or syrup, almond extract, ginger, orange zest (if using), and apple cider or juice. Whisk in the arrowroot until dissolved. Pour over the pears and apples and set aside.

To make the topping: In a separate bowl combine the oats, flour, almonds, and salt. In another smaller bowl, whisk together the agave nectar or syrup, oil, and almond extract. Add the wet ingredients to the dry ingredients and fold to combine.

Sprinkle the topping over the fruit in the casserole and spread out evenly. Cover with foil and bake for 35 minutes. Remove the foil and bake for another 15 minutes, until the topping is crisp and lightly brown. Remove from the oven and let sit for 5 to 7 minutes to cool. Serve warm.

Makes 6 to 8 servings

Chocolate Chip Cookies

Your entire family will love these chewy, chocolaty cookies. Keep your cookie jar filled with them so your kids can grab a healthy treat on the go.

2 cups spelt flour or a mixture of oat and spelt flour

¾ cup rolled oats

½ cup chopped walnuts (optional)

I cup grain-sweetened chocolate chips

½ teaspoon sea salt

¾ teaspoon baking soda

⅛ teaspoon cinnamon

¼ teaspoon cardamom

½ cup agave nectar or maple syrup

⅔ cup heated coconut, avocado, or grapeseed oil

3 tablespoons water or almond milk

I teaspoon vanilla or almond extract

Preheat the oven to 350°F. Line a baking sheet with parchment paper.

In a large mixing bowl, combine the flour, oats, walnuts (if using), chocolate chips, salt, baking soda, cinnamon, and cardamom. In a medium bowl, whisk together the agave nectar or syrup, oil, water or almond milk, and extract. Add the syrup mixture to the flour mixture and stir with a wooden spoon until combined. Refrigerate for 15 minutes.

Place the cookie dough by tablespoonsful on the prepared baking sheet. Bake for 10 to 12 minutes, or until golden brown. Remove and cool on a wire rack.

Makes approximately 3 dozen cookies

ACKNOWLEDGMENTS

I'd like to start out by saying that this book would not exist without Maggie Greenwood-Robinson, PhD. Her expertise and judgment shaped this book from the very beginning. She managed to turn my blogs, articles, chat room conversations, Facebook fan page–notes, interviews, and seminars into a comprehensive, streamlined synopsis of everything I've ever written, spoken about, and believed in. She is the consummate pro who held my hand throughout the process of creating my first book. Thank you, Maggie!

The funny flair for fitness goes to Fifer. The spark that ignited the idea of a Tony Horton book was Lara Ross. Lara was smart enough to introduce me to Barbara Lowenstein of Lowenstein Associates, who (after a little prodding) had the guts to represent a first-time author with the crazy idea that people might actually want an honest way of getting fit and healthy through hard work and clean eating.

Food and fitness are the one-two punch people need to create and sustain lasting change. Mark Briggs came to the rescue to help me develop the three-tiered workout program in *Bring It!* The Beginner's, Striver's, and Warrior's workouts came from a collaborative effort between Mark and me. His help and friendship during the creation of these routines has been invaluable. When it comes to making healthy food taste good, I had one main source: Missy Costello of KarmaChow.com fame. As many of you know, Missy cooks for me. In the old days, it was frozen food and a microwave that kept me alive. But then I rearranged my budget and put my money where my mouth is. You will prepare all your meals from this book with Missy's recipes. Lucky you! My editor, Julie Will, at Rodale Books is one of the nicest people on earth. Kind, patient, understanding, and always Will-ing to answer any and all of my naive first-time-writer questions. She made the final development process of this book a breeze. I'd also like to thank Zachary Greenwald, Amy King, Chris Rhoads, Emily Weber, and Marie Crousillat at Rodale for their invaluable efforts.

My life changed the day I met Mr. Carl Daikeler, Jon Congdon, and Ben Vandebunt. These fearless leaders of the direct marketing world are the main reasons why I'm no longer in debt up to my ears and living in a run-down apartment with a view of a convalescent home. Thanks also goes to the "Deal Makers," John Hendrickson and Jonathan Gelfand. Props to my Tuesday/Thursday morning crew: Scott Fifer, Erik Stolhanske, and Isaiah Mustafa. Without them, I'd just sleep in most mornings. To my Monday night crew: Veronica, Phil, Stasia, Steve, Neil, 5 Point Teddy, Greg, Sheila, Tom, Sean, Ashley, Michelle, Jay, and Tate. Our plyometric adventures keep my legs ready for the hills. Then there's the madmen who push me outside my comfort zone: Chuck Gaylord, Rami Ghandour, Brian Entman, Steve Holmsen, and, of course, Mr. Briggs. I can't forget the artists with a vision, who make me look good even when the lighting is bad: Nedd Farr and Mason Bendewald. And behind every good man there is a team of superwomen: Lily Moussa, who controls the chaos. Nicole Dunn, who expands my world. Dreya Weber, because she's such a badass! Suzanne Blankenship, my Beachbody Queen of Hearts. Susan Lucy's dedication and friendship. Three cheers go to supermom, camp coordinator, and my future cohost, Traci Morrow. And thanks to JuliAnne Forrest for all her help and hard work in DC and with my fitness camps.

This book would not exist were it not for the millions of Beachbody customers and coaches who decided, committed, and succeeded using my health and fitness programs. I also need to thank the members of Congress and all the men and women of the armed forces who use P90X, P90X Plus, and my One on One series as a way to stay ripped and ready. Thanks to Brigadier General Steven Shepro (Shep), and to Cousin David for the introduction and continued hard work.

Thanks to my family: Big Tone (that's my dad), Mary Beth, Larry, Andrew, Brian, rock-star sister Kit, Danny, Matthew, Liza, and Liam. Lastly, I'd like to thank my darling Shawna Marie Brannon. She's pure love and support—I love you, baby!

Endnotes

Chapter 5

1. Paoli, A., et al. 2010. "Effects of Three Distinct Protocols of Fitness Training on Body Composition, Strength, and Blood Lactate." *Journal of Sports Medicine and Physical Fitness* 50:43–51.

Chapter 8

1. Galper, D.I., et al. 2006. "Inverse Association between Physical Activity and Mental Health in Men and Women." *Medicine and Science in Sports and Exercise* 38:173–78.

Chapter 11

1. Krucoff, C. 1999. "Bodyworks: So You Want to Work Your Butt Off? Studies Show That the Top Techniques for Toning These Muscles Don't Require Special Gadgets." *Washington Post*, November 9.

Chapter 12

1. Tekur, P., et al. 2008. "Effect of Short-Term Intensive Yoga Program on Pain, Functional Disability, and Spinal Flexibility in Chronic Low Back Pain: A Randomized Control Study." *Journal of Complementary and Alternative Medicine* 14:637–44.

2. Gustafson, D.R., et al. 2009. "Adiposity Indicators and Dementia Over 32 Years in Sweden." *Neurology* 73:1559–66.

3. Norwood, J.T., et al. 2007. "Electromyographic Activity of the Trunk Stabilizers during Stable and Unstable Bench Press." *Journal of Strength and Conditioning Research* 21:343–47.

4. American Alliance for Health, Physical Education, Recreation, and Dance. 2001. "New Equipment Does Not Enhance Abdominal Exercises." *Journal of Physical Education, Recreation, and Dance*, August 1.

Chapter 14

1. Bray, G.A., et al. 2004. "Consumption of High-Fructose Corn Syrup in Beverages May Play a Role in the Epidemic of Obesity." *American Journal of Clinical Nutrition* 79:537–43.

2. Krilanovich, N.J. 2004. "Fructose Misuse, the Obesity Epidemic, the Special Problems of the Child, and a Call to Action." *American Journal of Clinical Nutrition* 80:1446–47.

3. Swithers, S.E., and Davidson, T.L. 2008. "A Role for Sweet Taste: Calorie Predictive Relations in Energy Regulation by Rats." *Behavioral Neuroscience* 122:161–73.

Chapter 15

1. Katcher, H.I., et al. 2008. "The Effects of a Whole Grain-Enriched Hypocaloric Diet on Cardiovascular Disease Risk Factors in Men and Women with Metabolic Syndrome." *American Journal of Clinical Nutrition* 87:79–90.
2. Childs, M.T., et al. 1990. "Effects of Shellfish Consumption on Lipoproteins in Normolipidemic Men." *American Journal of Clinical Nutrition* 51:1020–27.

Chapter 16

1. Fairfield, K.M., et al. 2002. "Vitamins for Chronic Disease Prevention in Adults: Scientific Review." *Journal of the American Medical Association* 287:3116–26.
2. Baser, K.H. 2008. "Biological and Pharmacological Activities of Carvacrol and Carvacrol Bearing Essential Oils." *Current Pharmaceutical Design* 14:3106–19.
3. Freedland, S.J., and Aronson, W.J. 2009. "Dietary Intervention Strategies to Modulate Prostate Cancer Risk and Prognosis." *Current Opinion in Urology* 19:263–67.

Chapter 17

1. King, A.C., et al. 1997. "Moderate-Intensity Exercise and Self-Rated Quality of Sleep in Older Adults: A Randomized Controlled Trial." *Journal of the American Medical Association* 277:32–7.
2. Buxton, O.M., et al. 2009. "Association of Sleep Adequacy with More Healthful Food Choices and Positive Workplace Experiences among Motor Freight Workers." *American Journal of Public Health* 99 Supplement 3:S636–43.

Index

Boldface page references indicate photographs. <u>Underscored</u> references indicate boxed text.